THE
A TO Z
BOOK OF
AGING

Live Long Live Well

MICHAEL P. EARNEY

ISBN-13: 978-1-956581-36-2 HB

Cover design and artwork by Michael P. Earney
Cover: "Off into the Sunset" colored pencil, by Michael P. Earney

Edited by Kate O'Donnell

ERIN GO BRAGH
Publishing

Canyon Lake, TX
www.ErinGoBraghPublishing.com

Acknowledgments

Thanks to the North family.

Thanks to Kate O'Donnell for suggesting aging as an A to Z book.

Thanks to Kathleen's Graphics for designing the interior.

Thanks and credits for the images used: BruceBlaus/Nick 163, Vincent van Gogh, Drugwatch.com, Blausen 0592, Merck Manuals, Etsy, Dreamtimes, Netmeds, Freepik, Mike Delima-O fashionnews.com, Prexels.com, Robin Higgins, Julia Bayly, Cape Cod Health News, TeachMeSurgery, Pixabay-MorShani, Pexels, CartoonStock, Anna Shvets, Cottonbro Studios, and Polina Tankilevitch.

Tomorrow

Tomorrow never comes.
Yesterday's tomorrow is today,
while tomorrow is tomorrow.
Whatever plans that you may have,
don't put them off until tomorrow.
Those 24 hours may not seem long,
but it's another day that will have gone,
another month, another year, another decade—
and now it seems you need a maid,
a driver, someone to see your bills are paid—
and where did I put that darned hearing aid?
Still, don't let's get all wrapped up in sorrow.
For, after all, there's still tomorrow.

Michael Earney
2024

Introduction

"Middle age is when you go to bed at night and hope you feel better in the morning. Old age is when you go to bed at night and hope you wake up in the morning."

—*Groucho Marx*

Whether animal or vegetable, the expected life cycle is this: We're born, we live, grow old, and die. But this is not true for the majority. In fact, many die in the womb, die at birth, die of starvation; we are struck by some killer disease, killed in an accident, a natural disaster, or a war; some commit suicide. Or as happens too often these days, we are in the wrong place at the wrong time and succumb to a random act of violence Those who manage to live a long life can also end in one of these ways or may simply die of old age. How old depends on any number of factors, including where and under what conditions one has lived, one's genetics, attitude, and just plain luck. There is no one way to reach old age, but one or another of the factors listed in this A to Z can play a role in determining whether or not we live a long life and if that life is healthy or plagued with pain and suffering.

Consider location: Petrochemical plants, usually located in areas predominantly housing people of color, produce toxic emissions that harm the community, the environment, and local wildlife- but permits for such facilities are continually issued. Coal-fired power plants routinely dump wastewater laced with lead, mercury, arsenic, and other toxins into our waterways. Cancer-causing chemicals are all around us. In the United States, thousands of children develop asthma every year due to traffic-related pollution. Multiply that number in far more polluted cities around the world. The list of health hazards grows daily as environmental problems increase, threatening the lives of more people, of wildlife, and of the planet we call home. And the list goes on. Preventable infectious diseases make up 6 of the top 10 causes of death in low-income countries. In 2021, 619,000 people died of malaria, 90 percent of them in Africa. Addiction to tobacco, alcohol, and other harmful drugs can shorten your life. Think, too, about the kinds of foods you eat: The longest-lived people eat a plant-based diet. Organically grown foods are obviously better for you than foods laced with chemicals. Stress at work, in the home, or due to any number of the conditions of everyday life—has negative health effects. The genes handed down from your ancestors can influence your chance of developing certain illnesses. If you're lucky, you'll have good genes rather than bad. And finally, how we choose to cope with problems affects our bodies and our minds.

Nevertheless, and despite all the odds, people do live into old age. And no matter the circumstances, how we cope is up to us. Whether living as a hermit in a cave or as a patient in a nursing home surrounded by loving, caring helpers, our attitude will have a lot to do with how we experience old age. Professor Li Chung Yun said his secret to a long life was this: *Keep a quiet heart, sit like a tortoise, walk sprightly like a pigeon, and sleep like a dog.*

August 2025

Father William

"You are old Father William," the young man said,
"And your hair has become very white;
And yet you incessantly stand on your head—
Do you think at your age, it is right?"

"In my youth." Father William replied to his son,
"I feared it might injure the brain;
But now that I'm perfectly sure I have none,
Why, I do it again and again."

"You are old," said the youth, "as I mentioned before,
And have grown most uncommonly fat;
Yet you turned a back-somersault in at the door—
Pray, what is the reason for that?"

"In my youth," said the sage, as he shook his grey locks,
"I kept all my limbs very supple
By the use of this ointment—one shilling the box—
Allow me to sell you a couple?"

"You are old," said the youth, "and your jaws are too weak
For anything tougher that suet;
Yet you finished the goose, with the bones and the beak—
Pray, how do you manage to do it?"

"In my youth," said his father, "I took to the law,
And argued each case with my wife;
And the muscular strength which it gave to my jaw,
Has lasted the rest of my life."

"You are old," said the youth, "one would hardly suppose
That your eye was as steady as ever;
Yet you balanced an eel on the end of your nose—
What made you so awfully clever?"

"I have answered three questions and that is enough,"
Said his father, "don't give yourself airs!
Do you think I can listen all day to such stuff?
Be off, or I'll kick you down stairs!"

—Lewis Carroll, *Alice's Adventures in Wonderland*

A is for Arthritis

Normal Joint

Muscle

Cartilage

Tendon

Bone

Joint Capsule

Synovium

Synovial Fluid

Bone

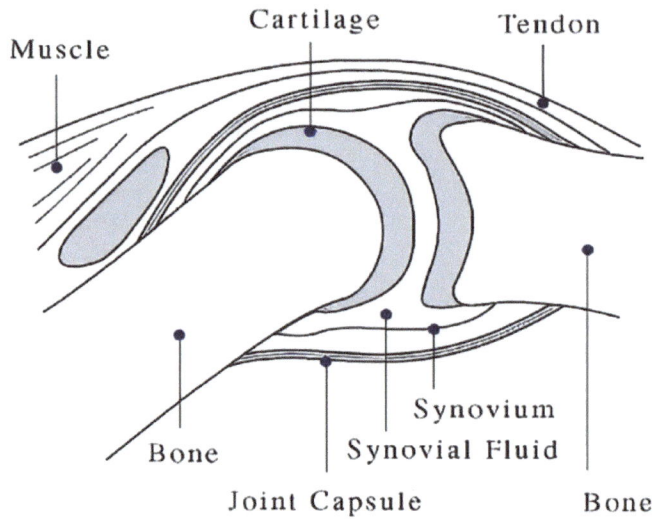

Joint Affected by Rheumatoid Arthritis

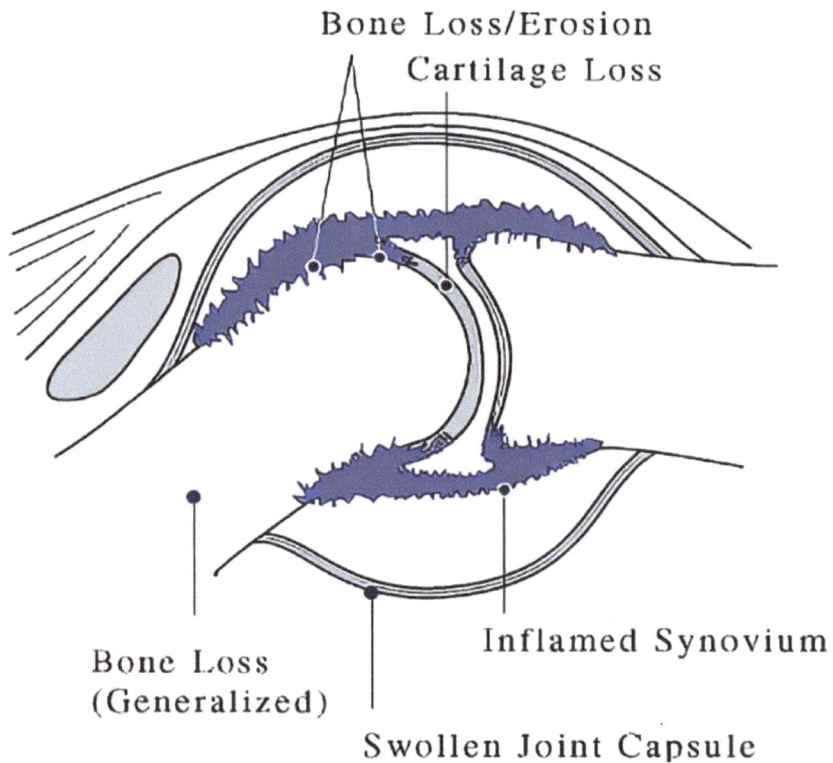

Bone Loss/Erosion

Cartilage Loss

Bone Loss (Generalized)

Inflamed Synovium

Swollen Joint Capsule

"Well, my friends are gone and my hair is gray, I ache in the places where I used to play."

—Leonard Cohen, *Tower of Love*

A is for **Arthritis**. It's not unusual to have aches and pains, especially as you grow older, but if the pain is right at the joint of two bones, you could be developing arthritis. According to the Centers for Disease Control and Prevention (CDC), arthritis is the leading cause of disability in the US, affecting some 58.8 million people. As you age there's a good chance you will become one of them. So what can you do about it? First, it will help to know what kind of arthritis it is. There are over 100 joint and surrounding tissue conditions that fall under the name of arthritis. Gout is one; psoriatic arthritis, which occurs in people who have psoriasis, is another. In rheumatoid arthritis, the problem tends to be symmetrical, affecting both wrists, both knees, and so on, the mechanisms that normally protect the body instead begin to attack the joint tissues. Osteoarthritis, the most common form, may be caused by trauma or may be just a sign of the wear and tear of old age.

The bad news is there's no cure for arthritis. The good news is you can do things to relieve the pain. Losing weight is one. For every 10 pounds you gain, your knees feel 30 pounds more pressure. Also, stay active! Engage in low-impact exercises like swimming or cycling but use a stationary bike or ride leisurely through the park. Don't go mountain biking! Topical creams or ointments may help (CBD is becoming a favored treatment), as can certain drugs, although these may harm other parts of the body. Braces, splints, injections, and even surgery may be the answer. Knee, hip, and shoulder replacements are becoming increasingly routine. As always, you must decide whether the benefits outweigh the risks. An experimental treatment using nanoparticles is showing good results, and according to Rice University biologist Vicky Yao, taking care of your teeth might help prevent arthritis!

If you see a bunch of old folks in the park doing weird, slow, coordinated movements, join them! Qi gong, tai chi, yoga: people have been doing these movements for centuries because they work! If you aren't in a position to go to a park, take up the practice at home. A yoga mat under your bare feet feels nice, and you can learn the moves from a video or on YouTube. Establish a routine of practicing one of these tried and trusted activities. T'ai Chi Ch'uan comes from 12th-century China; a much newer version known as Tai chi che or chih, called the *joy of movement*, is easy to learn and practice. Those with Parkinson's disease or other disabilities that keep them off their feet can do seated tai chi or chair yoga. Indeed, tai chi has been found to slow the progress of Parkinson's and to lower patients' medication needs.

Cool Fact: The first public performance of tai chi in the United States was given at the Museum of Modern Art in New York by the dancer Sophia Delza in 1954. Delza taught tai chi and wrote the first English language book on the subject. She died at age 92 in 1996.

What other aging problem starts with A?

B

is for Brain

"By the time you're 80 yrs. old you've learned everything. You just have to remember it."

—*George Burns*

B is for **Brain**. What is the brain, anyway? In the average human, it weighs about 3 pounds and is made up mostly of fat; the rest is water, proteins, carbohydrates, and salt. The brain controls our thoughts, memory, emotions, vision, breathing, motor skills, touch, temperature, hunger, and every process that regulates the body. (The Scarecrow in *The Wizard of Oz* would not have been able to *wish* he had a brain if he didn't already have one.) How does it do all that? In the cranium (the dome of the skull) there are 12 nerves: first the olfactory nerve, which allows you to smell; next the optic nerve, which lets you see; and so on. Only the first two nerves originate in the cranium; the brain stem is the source of the rest. All the cells that make up the brain are in constant communication through chemicals known as neurotransmitters. Glutamate, serotonin, and dopamine are some of those neurotransmitters, and too much or too little of any one of them is responsible for many of the problems of aging. As we age, communication between the transmitters breaks down. The amino acid taurine, which is naturally abundant in the body and is said to be the key to a long and healthy life, declines with age. Also the brain shrinks, blood flow may decrease, and inflammation from injuries and overuse of alcohol may affect aging.

Like the body, the brain needs exercise to stay healthy—and maintaining a healthy and active body also helps the brain. Diet has a role as well. The high number of centenarians in Okinawa and throughout Japan is thought to be due at least in part to their plant-based diet. Other factors include maintaining connections through generations of family, strong social networks, staying positive, and enjoying life. The older brain *can* change and adapt, it just takes longer than before. *Cognitive super-agers* are people in their 80s and 90s who have memory performance comparable to that of people 20 to 30 years younger. It's possible!

So use that lifetime of accumulated knowledge and experience to lighten your day. Talking about the past may bore some people, but it can also be a source of enlightenment and joy. Reminiscing may help to alleviate some of those "senior moments." There are also any number of cognitive games available to help keep your brain sharp, just as there are any number of brain-boosting supplements and pills to improve your memory, focus, concentration, and mood. Supplements can help but be sure to check reputable reviews before you lay out the big bucks: In 2021, the global anti-aging market was worth $37 billion. In his book *The Anti-Aging Manual*, Dr. Joseph B. Marion wrote: "If we are using 4–14% of our brain to live to 100, there may be a combination of nutrients that would enable us to utilize 30–50–100% more thinking power. Could the brain's power be stretched to perceive on a higher level and to live 200–300–500 years as more conscious beings?" I wonder…

Cool Fact: A study carried out by a Yale psychologist found that participants with a rosier perception of their aging lived 7.5 years longer than the less positive participants.

What other aging problem starts with B?

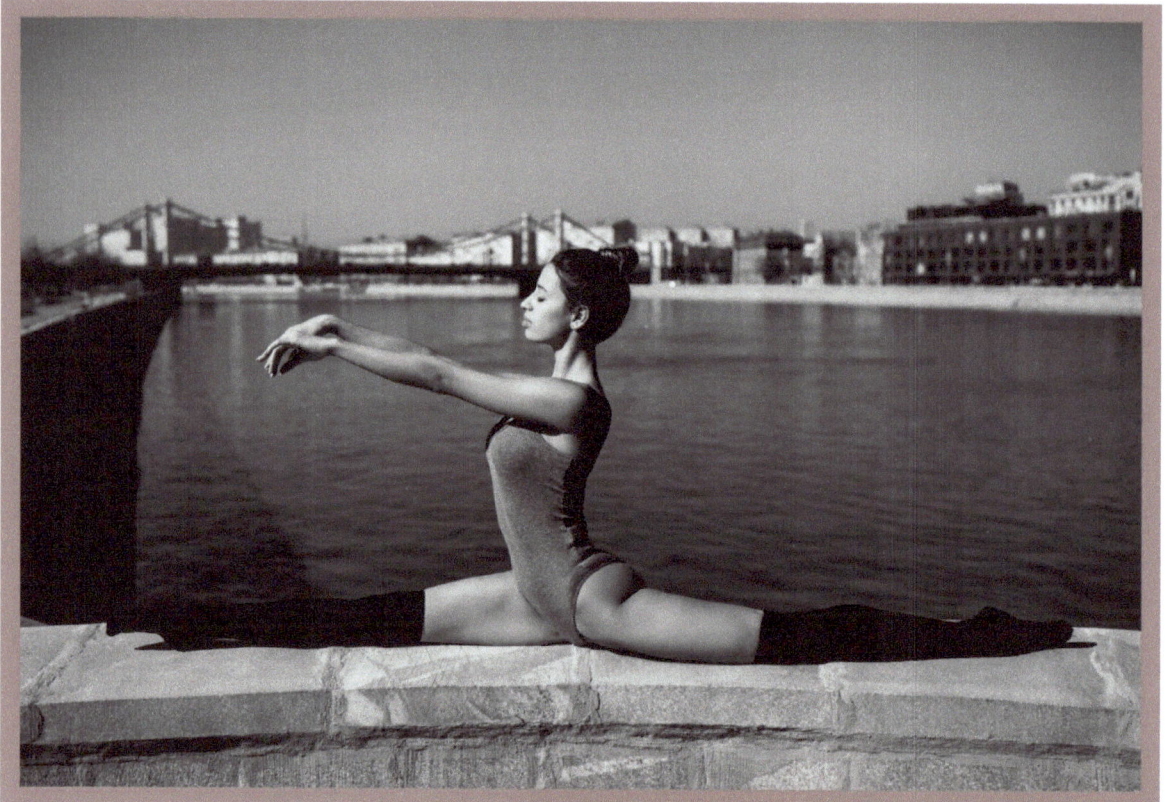

C

is for
Cramps

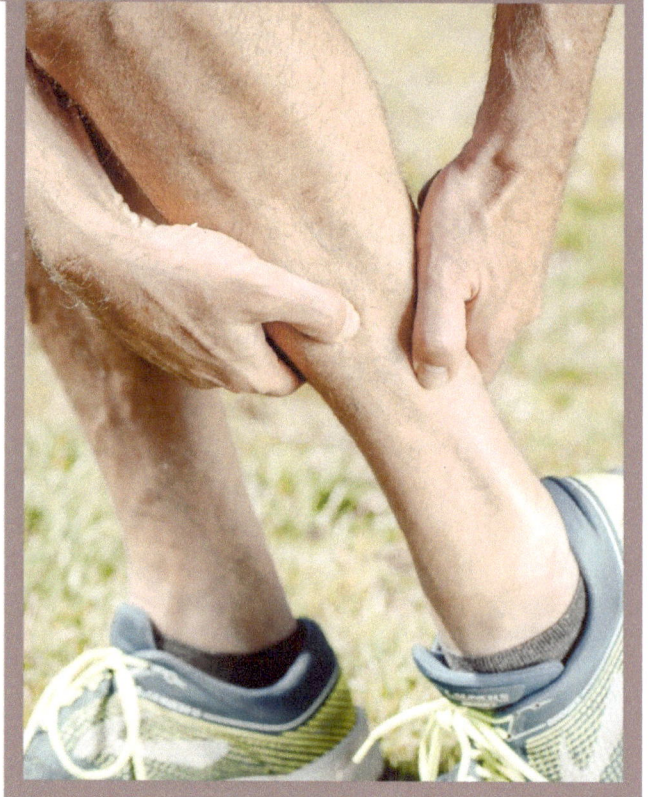

"You have to stay in shape. My grandmother started walking 5 miles a day when she was 60. She's 97 today and we have no idea where the hell she is."

—*George Carlin*

C is for **Cramps**. Stomach cramps, heart cramps, leg cramps, nocturnal cramps. Studies have shown that almost a third of adults over 60 and nearly half of adults over 80 suffer from them. There is a long list of vitamins, minerals, bioflavonoids, and electrolytes that are needed to avoid cramping. Without the minerals, the vitamins won't work. Luckily, most of the minerals and vitamins needed to stop cramps are found in the foods we eat if we have a well-balanced diet. Unfortunately, many of the foods we eat also contain enzymes that can cause cramping. "Forever chemicals" that we ingest also don't help. Too-strenuous physical activity and insufficient oxygen limit glucose burning, and the glucose then forms lactic acid that shuts down muscle contraction. The muscles then burn and cramp.

While the Charley horse is often associated with strenuous exercise, it can just as easily occur when you are peacefully sleeping. Those extremely painful nocturnal cramps can last a few seconds or several minutes. What to do? I have found that placing my foot on the cold floor helps. There are also many natural remedies. Calcium, phosphorous, potassium, magnesium, copper, and gold—traces of which are found in horsetail, alfalfa, raspberry, asparagus, and honey mixed with apple cider vinegar—all have been credited at different times with offering relief. But nocturnal leg cramps are caused by a different set of conditions than those causing other cramps, and professionals are still stumped as to what to do about them. Formulas concocted to fight cramps are usually based on magnesium, but not all magnesium is created equal. Magnesium glycinate is said to be the one to take right before bed, but none of the magnesium-based cures have been found to be effective for the aged. Caleb Treeze, an old Amish muscle tonic, is 100 percent guaranteed. It contains organic apple cider, vinegar, all-natural ginger, and garlic juice. Music, too, can relax cramping.

Fever-Tree tonic water, or any low-sodium tonic water containing quinine, has been found to help some people with muscle cramps, although *Men's Health* cites a study that found people taking quinine had a risk of dying before their time and it is no longer recommended due to some fatal reactions. Quinine is derived from the bark of the cinchona (chicona) tree, which is native to South America. It was transplanted to many parts of Africa, India, and China where malaria was thinning the ranks of European settlers. Malaria still affects an estimated 240 million people worldwide, causing 619,000 deaths yearly. Many malaria vaccines are being tested that show varying degrees of success.

Cool Fact: In the 18th century British soldiers in India took to drinking tonic water containing quinine to fight malaria. Because the tonic water was quite bitter, the soldiers started adding gin, and then lime or lemon, to combat the bitterness. Voila! The gin and tonic is born!

What other aging problems start with C?

D is for Depression

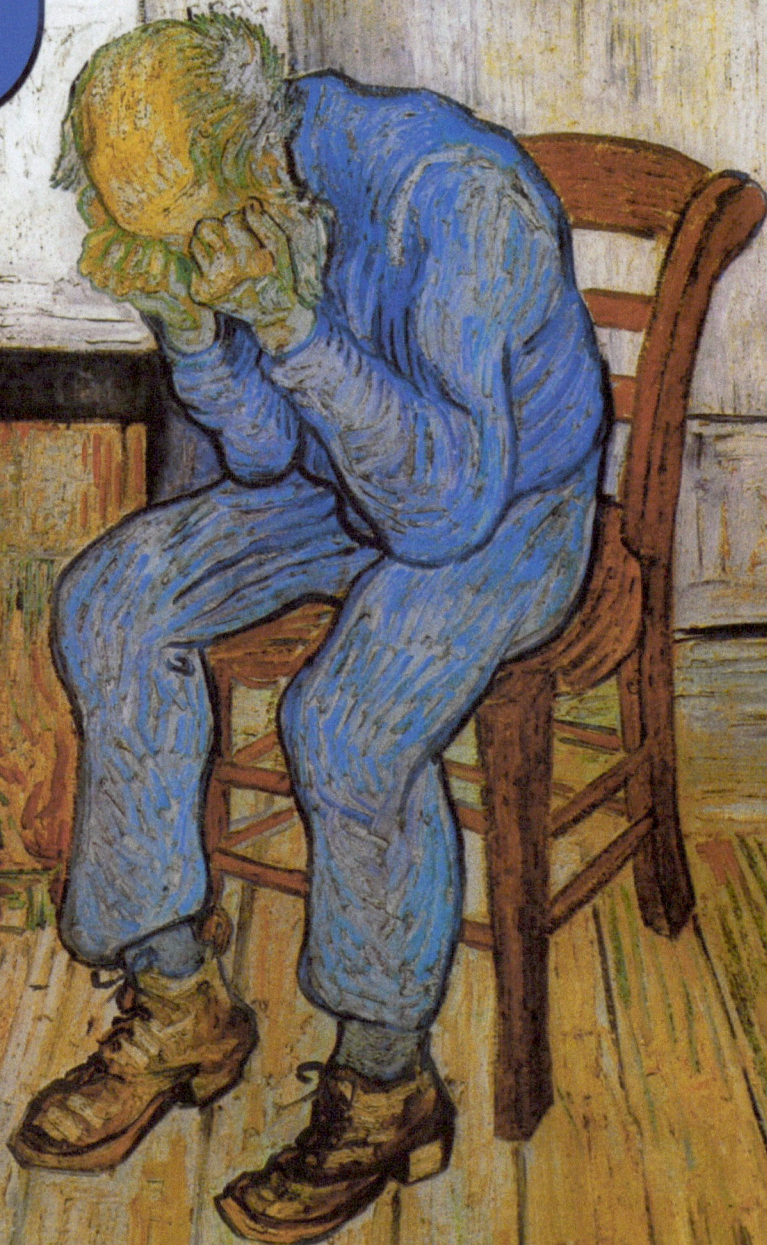

"Last year I was miserable and depressed. But this year I've turned things around. Now I'm depressed and miserable."

—Laffgaff.com

D is for **Depression**. Depression can hit anyone at any time. It is relatively common among children and adolescents, and its occurrence can continue into adulthood. Even if you have lived a reasonably happy life, the woes of old age can result in depression. Psychological factors can affect the very chemistry of our bodies. Low levels of cortisol, produced by stress, lead to feelings of weakness and tiredness; high levels can lead to weight gain. So exercise and healthful eating can lessen the effects of stress and depression. Remembering to drink sufficient amounts of water every day is important. And antidepressants prescribed by a professional may help, though they can have their downsides too, including weight gain. If depression gets too bad, and if suicidal thoughts ever occur, it's best to consult a therapist. This can be done online these days! If you have an internet connection, you can meet with a therapist in the privacy of your own home. Uncovering and releasing the inner pain could bring a lasting cure. And if you or anyone you know is having thoughts of suicide, please call 988.

Depression and body weight—either gain or loss—are often linked. Binge eating as a relief from feeling down does work temporarily, but it often leads to more depression over the extra weight gained or the inability to control the urge to eat. This negative spiral can lead to self-disgust and to choosing to be alone—which also has its downside. Conversely, some people lose weight when they are depressed. They have no appetite for food, no motivation to do the things they usually enjoy, like going out to eat with friends, or to do much of anything. When depression hits and you don't want to exercise, the endorphins and other chemicals released through exercise, which can improve one's your mood, are not released into the brain.

So, what if you are confined to bed or to a wheelchair, all your loved ones are gone, and you suffer great aches and pains? You have given up hope and have no desire to go on? That's the downward spiral that could lead you to a (hopefully) peaceful death! Yes, laugh! Laughter is a natural remedy for depression: it releases endorphins and raises their level in our brains. A hearty laugh activates the muscles of the abdomen similar to the way exercise does. Whatever physical and mental activities you can participate in will make a difference. The simple act of taking care of a plant or a pet, feeling like you are doing something useful, enjoying good company even if it's nonhuman, will make you more aware of what a beautiful and amazing world it is to be alive in.

Cool Fact: The list of comedians who battle depression is very long, and many have based their entire careers on making jokes about depression. Humor allows them to deal with subjects people don't like to talk about. They are making light of the dark.

What other aging problems start with D?

E is for Eyesight

1	E	1
2	YE	2
3	SAW	3
4	VIEW	4
5	OGLED	5
6	GLANCE	6

―――――――――――――

7	PERUSAL	7
8	OBSERVER	8

―――――――――――――

9	FOCALIZED	9
10	TRANSFIXED	10
11	OBSERVATION	11

The left eye said to the right eye, "Just between you and me, something smells."

—Anonymous

E is for **Eyesight**. The five sensory organs—the eyes, nose, ears, skin, and tongue—keep us aware of the world around us by sending messages to the brain. Losing any of these senses can range from bothersome to dangerous. Can you enjoy a meal if you can't taste it? Touch, aside from its sensual aspect, is necessary for our very survival. If you can't feel the heat of a boiling pot, serious injury can occur. Hearing loss is very common as one ages; luckily, hearing aids can alleviate much of this problem, unless one becomes totally deaf. There may be any number of things you would be happy to never smell again, but as with all the senses, *not* smelling something can be dangerous. And just imagine not smelling the spring flowers!

For many of us, losing our vision is perhaps the greatest worry. It's not uncommon for our eyesight to fade as we age. Blue light, to which we expose ourselves daily through television, fluorescent lights, computers, laptops, and cell phone screens, takes its toll. Glasses with an anti-glare coating and blue-light-filtering glasses are worth the investment if you spend a lot of time looking at screens—and who doesn't? As our aging sight deteriorates, we turn first to over-the-counter reading glasses, then to distance glasses so we can still drive. After that, we might progress to the three-way—read, drive, and see the signs in the store—glasses. Each visit to the optician can result in an upgrade in the lenses needed.

Diseases of the eye are a different matter. If you're experiencing macular degeneration, cataracts, or glaucoma, in which the optic nerve at the back of the eye is damaged and causes pain, nausea, red eye, and blurry vision—you should go to your doctor or to an emergency room right away. If you look online, you can find any number of pills, shots, and injections that claim to save you from Lasik surgery and other eye problems, but don't fall for the snake oil salesmen! (They haven't gone away; they've just moved to Google search.) One surgical intervention that's become more popular is the removal of cloudy cataract lenses and replacement with clear artificial lenses—but make sure your ophthalmologist recommends these. There are also things you can do to keep your eyes healthy. Eye exercises are a good addition to your daily exercise routine, especially if you sit in front of the computer for hours on end. Blinking, eye-rolling, focus shifting, and palming can help alleviate dry eye and are good for your eyes generally. There are books and courses on eye exercises available, with routines lasting from 35 minutes to as long as 4 hours. And some are free! Eye massage is also another good habit to get into.

Cool Fact: British jazz musician Sir George Shearing was blind from birth but learned to play piano. As a teenager, he joined a band of blind musicians. Ray Charles lost his eyesight at age 7. At school, he learned to read and compose music in Braille. Stevie Wonder, blind almost from birth, started playing piano at age 5 and was 11 when he signed with a Motown label. At 13 he became the youngest musician to hit the Billboard Hot 100. And at age 38, in 1989, Wonder was the youngest living person ever inducted into the Rock and Roll Hall of Fame.

What other aging problems start with E?

F is for Facelift

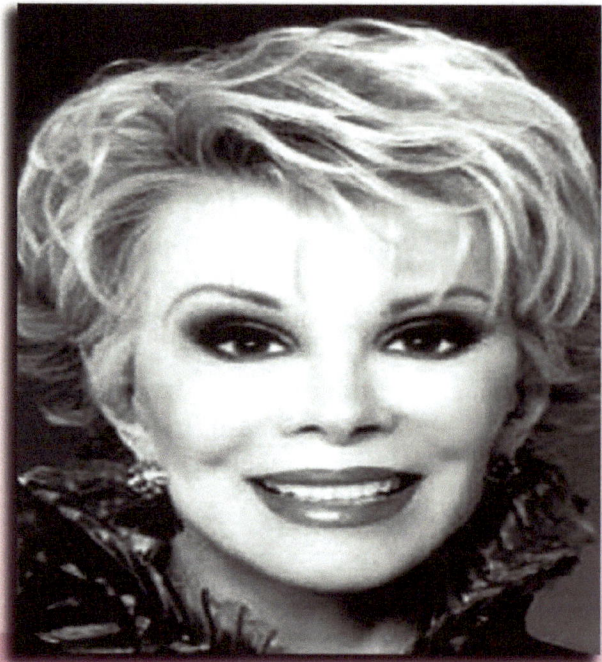

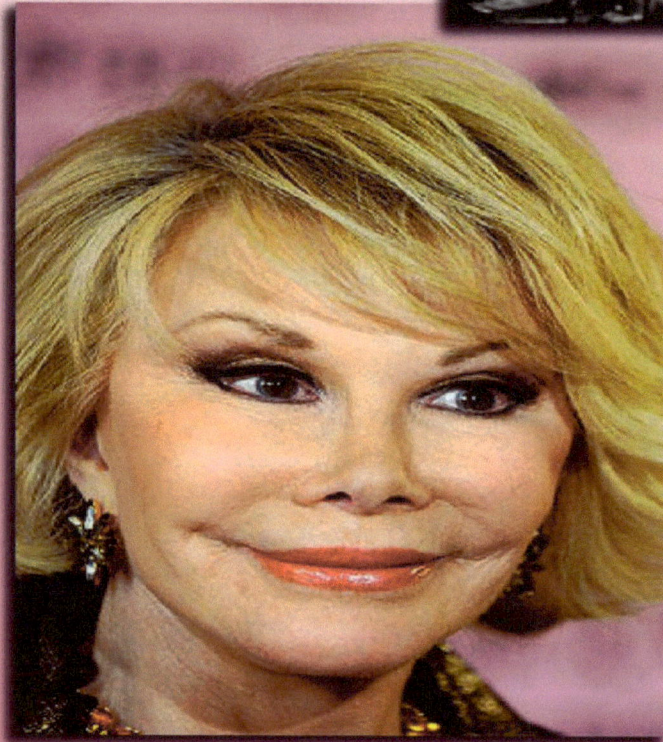

Cosmetic surgery used to be such a taboo subject.
Now you can talk about Botox and nobody raises an eyebrow.

—Upjoke.com

F is for **Facelift**. If you are a movie star or a model, or if your interaction with the public requires you to appear young, healthy, beautiful, or virile, keeping the appearance of youth may tempt you to get some kind of cosmetic surgery. Plastic surgery has been around for centuries: the first facelift we know of was performed in 1901, when a Polish aristocrat asked a German surgeon if he could lift her cheeks and the corners of her mouth. The surgeon accomplished this by removing two elliptical pieces of skin around the woman's ear areas. Sewing the edges back together raised and tightened the skin.

In 1907 the first textbook on facelifting, *The Correction of Featured Imperfections*, was published by Charles Miller of Chicago. In 1916 another German surgeon and former sculptor(!), Dr. Erich Lexer, did a procedure in which the facial skin was lifted from the underlying fat layer and pulled tighter. For the next 60 years, this was the predominant type of facelift. It tended to be called the "wind tunnel look," as the skin looked so extremely tight and taut. In the 1970s the SMAS (superficial muscular aponeurotic system) technique was developed. This involved deeper incisions so that deeper tissue could be adjusted and sutured. Between 1981 and 1990, coronal incisions were being made in order to lift the skin over the skeletal structure. Dr. Sam Hamra developed the "deep plane facelift," which targeted those lower tissue layers. Facial cosmetic surgery continues to be refined to reduce scarring, accelerate healing time, and minimize severe side effects. And, of course, to make you look young again.

Although you'll see pictures of celebrities whose surgery has gone disastrously wrong, 70 percent of patients report being satisfied with their cosmetic surgery results 12 years later. Men and women who don't smoke and have healthy healing responses are the best candidates for such surgery, but the potential risks are substantial: accumulation of fluid under the skin, bleeding, infection, nerve-related complications, scarring, skin discoloration, asymmetrical results—on top of all the other risks associated with major surgery. Today there are neck-lift and eyelid-lift surgeries. While you're about it, you might as well get breast implants, too. But even these, like Botox and cosmetic filler injections, don't last forever. Then again, how long do you want to retain that youthful look, anyway? For some, it bolsters the sense of self-worth and is a badge of resisting the ravages of old age. But nothing, dear reader, is going to stop the advance and ultimate triumph of age. Exercise, a good diet, good genes, good luck, and healthy living are still the best way to deal with aging. They won't erase the wrinkles, though!

Cool Fact: Comedian Joan Rivers (1933–2014), well known for her cosmetic surgery and her jokes about it, left an archive of 65,000 cross-referenced jokes. One of the items cataloged under "OLD" is this: "I'm so old, the first time I had sex was in the back of a chariot."

What other old age problems start with F?

G

is for **Gallbladder**

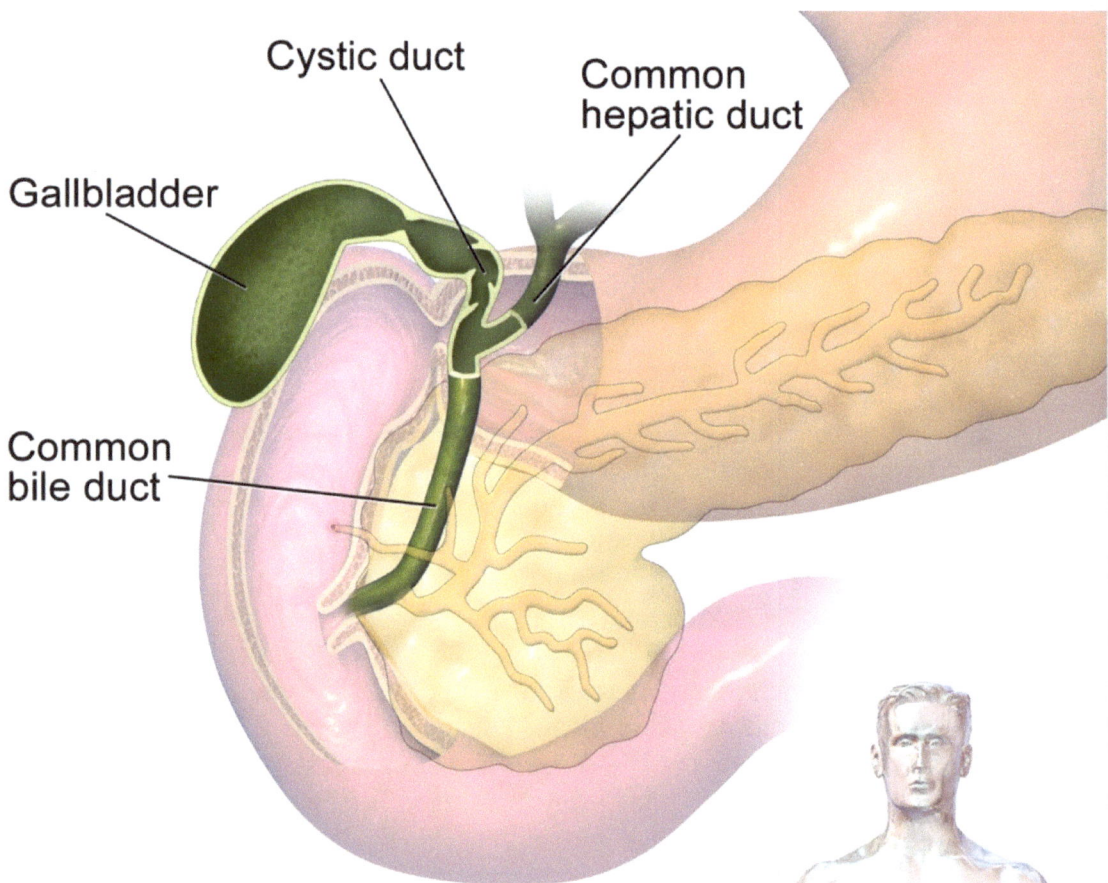

Cystic duct

Common
hepatic duct

Gallbladder

Common
bile duct

The Gallbladder

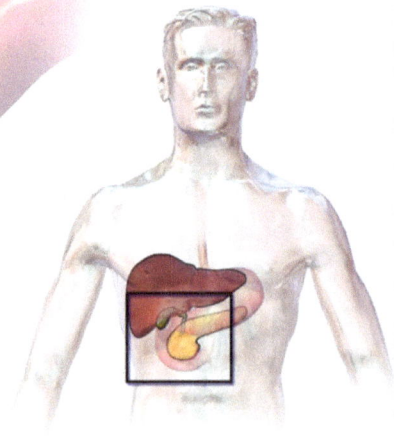

Poster seen on a Gallstone Specialist's office wall, "This Too Shall Pass."

—*Cartoonstock*

G is for **Gallbladder**. The marvelous gallbladder works away in the body, fulfilling its duties just like all the rest of our equipment with no fuss, drawing no attention—until it doesn't. That's if you have a normal gallbladder. In fact, you can have 2 or 3 gallbladders, each draining separately into the cystic duct or sharing a common branch into the cystic duct. The location of the gallbladder can also vary, being behind, above, or even inside the liver. There is also an anatomical variation known as a Phrygian cap.

Bile or gall—hence the organ's name—flows from the liver into the gallbladder, where it is concentrated 3- to 10-fold before being released into the stomach to mix with pancreatic acid and digest whatever it is you just ate. No surprise, then, that what you eat will affect the functioning of the gallbladder. Vegetables, fruits, and greens provide fiber. Lysine, an essential amino acid that regulates the gallbladder, is not produced by the human body but it is found in animal products: meat, fish, dairy, and eggs. If your gallbladder is removed for medical reasons, the liver steps in and retains the bile to release as needed, though you may suffer indigestion as a result. Certain vegetables, including artichokes, increase gallbladder secretions and help to counter digestive problems. A number of herbs, such as parsley, are also said to be useful for the functioning of the gallbladder. Choose carefully, though! Unfortunately, we have little control over much of what we take into our bodies. Pesticides, herbicides, and preservatives are virtually unavoidable and adversely affect our digestion. If your liver isn't working right due to poor diet, alcoholism, or other causes, the gallbladder is going to have a hard time doing its job, which can lead to all kinds of health problems that are often blamed on "old age." Simply improving your diet can eliminate some of these.

Gallstones form in the gallbladder when the bile is saturated with cholesterol or bilirubin, elements that are normally excreted in the bile and urine. Luckily, most gallstones don't cause problems and either remain in the gallbladder or pass through your system with little more than a "colicky" pain. But if the stones block the gallbladder, the disease cholecystitis may develop. Various natural remedies have been used to dissolve the stones: sesame seed oil, lecithin, burdock, and calamus among them—and the last of these was also placed near the door by the ancient Chinese to counter evil influences. Joking aside, gallbladder issues and gallstones are a prevalent cause of hospitalization: 60 to 70 percent of the elderly have cholesterol or calcium gallstones, and gallstone disease is the most common digestive disorder in the U.S.

Cool Fact: The Phrygian cap, or liberty cap, was worn in antiquity by a number of peoples ranging from Eastern Europe to Persia. During the American Revolution and the later French Revolution, the cap came to symbolize freedom and liberty. Made of wool or soft leather, it was a conical hat with a flipped-over tip. Early Christian art often depicted the Three Wise Men wearing Phrygian caps.

What other old age problem starts with G?

H

is for Hearing

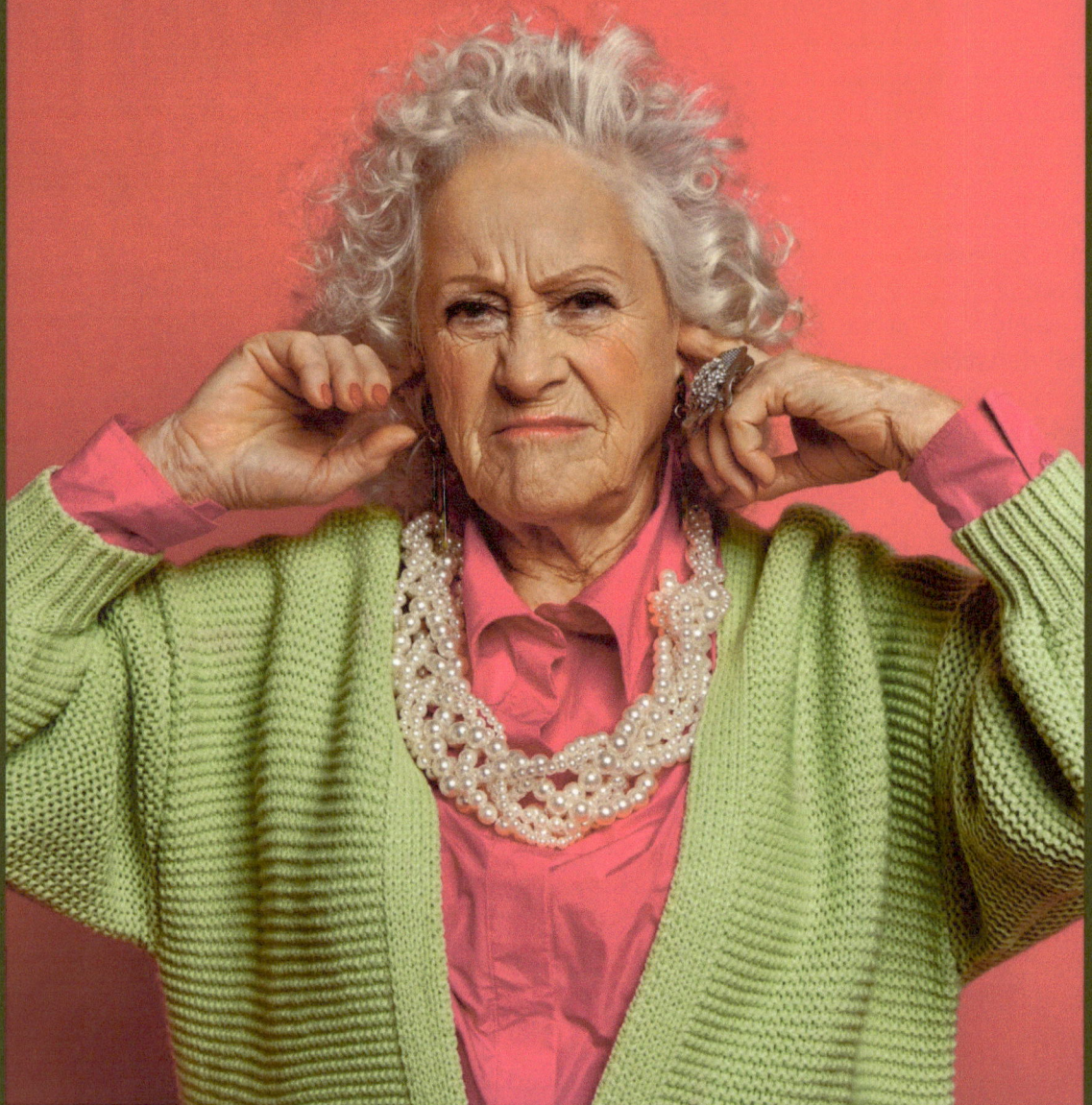

The host asks the dinner guest. "Have you had sufficient?" "You say you've been fishing?"
"No, no, I said have you had plenty?" "You caught twenty!"
"No, you old fool." "Oh no, you broke your pole." The host gives up.

—Anonymous.

H is for **Hearing**. Another common ailment associated with aging is hearing loss. Over a lifetime, any number of factors might contribute to the loss of hearing. Exposure to loud noises should be avoided, but unfortunately, we don't always realize that until it's too late. When I did my National Service, I was required to fire guns, and no form of hearing protection was provided. (Would earplugs have blown the national defense budget?) All kinds of products are sold that have unacceptable noise levels; users are expected to protect themselves. Especially when we're young, we don't think of such things. Too often, no one warns us.

The Occupational Safety and Health Administration (OSHA) requires employers to provide hearing protection, but some companies find OSHA standards to be over-burdensome and others simply ignore them. If your inner ear or auditory nerve is damaged due to exposure to loud noise, disease, or genetic variations, you will definitely need professional assistance. Otosclerosis is a form of abnormal bone growth within the ear that can lead not only to hearing loss but also to tinnitus and can affect one's balance. Ear wax buildup can also affect our hearing. Don't use a Q-Tip! There are any number of ear wax drops and removal kits. Some are better than others.

No matter what the cause, hearing loss is something you can expect to experience as you age. You may need hearing aids and hearing protection. Hearing aids come in all sizes, shapes, applications, and costs. They don't restore normal hearing, but they do amplify sound. The primary types of hearing aids are the CIC (completely in the canal), the ITC (in the canal), the ITE (in the ear), and the BTE (behind the ear). The CIC is the smallest and least visible and is less likely to pick up wind noise, but it has small, short-life batteries that may not be rechargeable. The ITC has more features, longer life, and rechargeable batteries, as does the ITE. BTEs have a tube connecting the aid to an earpiece that fits in the ear canal. There are other types that feature the receiver in the canal (RIC), the receiver in the ear (RIE), and the open fit (OF). All of these hearing aids are susceptible to earwax clogging.

Make sure your device comes with a trial period and is returnable, as it may take a while to decide which is the one for you. And get one with a warranty! Hearing aids are relatively expensive, although over-the-counter versions are becoming more easily available and less pricey. But no hearing aid lasts forever, and Medicare *still* doesn't cover the cost for adults. As a last resort, there's always the ear trumpet, as seen in old illustrations and movies!

Cool Fact: There are more than 300 different sign languages used around the world, each employing hands, eyes, facial expressions, and movements to communicate. Although most prominently used by people who are hearing impaired, they are also used by hearing people. ASL (American Sign Language) is the first language of more than a million people.

What other old age problem starts with H?

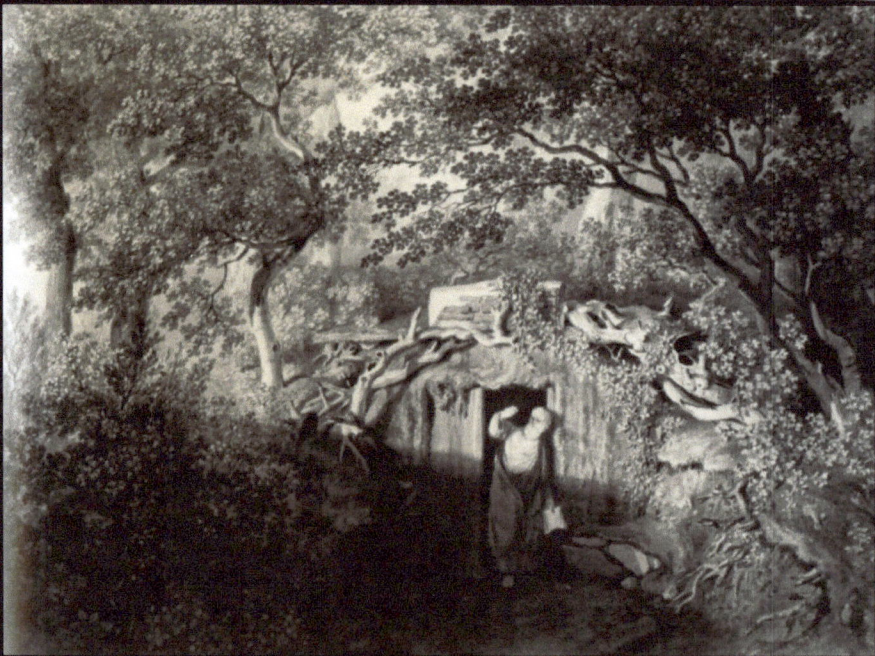

is for Isolation

"Getting old is like climbing a mountain;
you get out of breath, but the view is much better."

—*Ingrid Bergman*

I is for **Isolation**. If you grew up in a large, close, loving family that celebrated holidays together and maintained lifelong connections with friends and relatives, you may have never known isolation. Even so, as we age our families disperse, members die, friends die, and some become confined to a wheelchair, to their bed, or to an institution of some kind. This may happen to you. Being unable to get around due to failing eyesight, difficulty communicating due to hearing loss, or the simple lack of energy and motivation all contribute to increased isolation. Loneliness and isolation are not the same, but one can lead to the other.

Living like a hermit, far from the madding crowd, self-sufficient, communing with nature, raising a garden, keeping a few animals, listening to the birds and the wind in the trees, walking the hills: that's one kind of isolation. Solitary confinement is another. In prisons all over the world, solitary confinement is used as a form of punishment. An incarcerated person is shut in a single cell with few or no amenities for up to 22 to 23 hours a day and for periods ranging from days to years. (When British serial killer Robert Maudsley reached age 64, he had spent 49 of those years in prison, nearly 45 of them in solitary, setting a "world record.")

Solitary confinement, especially long-term, can have harmful and lasting psychological effects on the prisoner. It is widely considered a form of torture, sometimes used to extract a confession. Even the sort of isolation one experiences in ordinary life can have a deleterious effect on mental health. The isolation that too many experience as a factor of getting old carries the risk of heart disease, depression, and cognitive decline. Loneliness biases our thinking and makes us less likely to connect with others, to trust them, or to want to engage. Loneliness and depression can affect us even when we do have access to others but choose to withdraw and disengage from those around us and end up spiraling downwards into solitude and silence. Retreating into memories and anthropomorphizing your pet are not recommended, as they can make it increasingly difficult to interact with others.

Zoom meetings, video chats, and simple telephone calls can help to dispel the isolation. While not perfect, these are important ways to keep in touch with friends and family. As the Bill Withers song says, "We all need somebody to lean on."

Online resources such as Elder Care Locators and Expand Your Circle: Prevent Isolation and Loneliness as You Age can be useful, as can the NIH (National Institutes of Health), which offers a number of Social Isolation and Loneliness Outreach toolkits.

Cool Fact: Volunteers for an experiment conducted in Switzerland took psilocybin, the active ingredient in magic mushrooms; later, they reported feeling less socially excluded, and their brain scans showed decreased activity in the areas that process painful social experiences.

What other aging problems start with I?

J is for Joints

What did one bone say to another bone? Let's meet up and share a joint.
—*Upjokes.com*

J is for **Joints**. Not those kinds of joints! No, we're talking about the ones that squeak, creak, click, pop, or lock whenever you sit, stand, bend, or try to pick something up. Yes, *those* joints. Even if you were never an athlete, played contact sports, or fell down the stairs, your old, aching joints will feel like you did all those things yesterday.

Bone density and mass are lost as we age, and our dietary habits can make things worse. Falls are more likely as we get older, and weak bones are prone to fracture as calcium, other minerals, and amino acids diminish. The most common cause of joint pain is arthritis, of which there are more than 100 types. But ailments such as viruses, bursitis, tendonitis, and an infection that can be a side effect of cancer treatment can cause joint pain. The cartilage that covers the surface of our bones and cushions them against impact degrades over time, and bones start to grind on each other. You may have to learn a whole new set of movements to eat, sleep, stand, and walk without being in constant pain. But if you restrict movement to avoid the pain, your joints will only atrophy and the muscles weaken more, so you must learn ways to relieve pain and strengthen muscles to prevent them from shortening.

Massage, acupuncture, and physical therapy can help. Braces or splints can support movement: correctional splints for motion and resting splints for use at night. Elastic bandages can support your knees. *How* you sleep—from your pillow to your sleeping position—can also affect your joints. Heating pads, warm baths, showers, or ice packs provide relief for swollen joints. Watch your posture and don't slouch. Be aware of simple adjustments: keep your back against the back of the chair or seat, whether driving or writing; keep your knees at the same height or slightly lower than your hips, and your feet flat on the floor. The type of shoes you wear, too, has an impact.

Eat healthy, give up processed foods and saturated fats, and don't smoke! To maintain the calcium in your joints, cut down on soda pop, coffee, and alcohol. Carbonated soft drinks contain high levels of phosphoric acid, which increases our blood acidic levels; in response, the body pulls calcium from our bones, lowering bone mass. Supplements containing collagen claim to rebuild cartilage and strengthen joints, but their true health benefits are unknown. Collagen is the most abundant protein in the body, but we produce less as we age, and its quality decreases. Trials in cartilage replenishment are underway, but in the meantime eating a healthy diet seems to be the best way to maintain healthy joints and avoid osteoporosis. And while we're on the subject of joints, the cannabis derivative CBD is now widely available and legal as edible gummies and in other forms. It may offer relief from pain and inflammation, lower stress levels, and even give you a good night's sleep.

Cool Fact: Chicharones—pork rinds, baked or fried in avocado oil—provide protein and collagen. Sometimes made using chicken, mutton, or beef, they are popular throughout the world in various forms and under different names. In the United Kingdom, they are known as "pork scratchings."

What other aging problems start with J?

K is for Kidney

Renal cortex

Hilum

Renal artery

Renal vein

Renal medulla

Renal papilla

Renal pyramids

Renal pelvis

Renal columns

Ureter

Major calyx

Minor calyx

Fibrous capsule

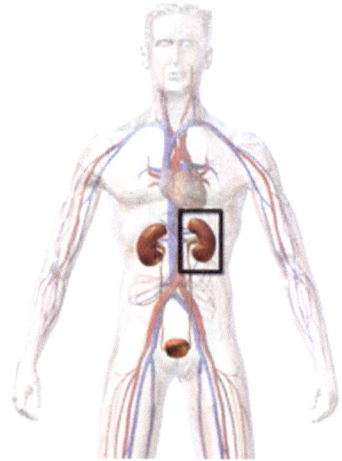

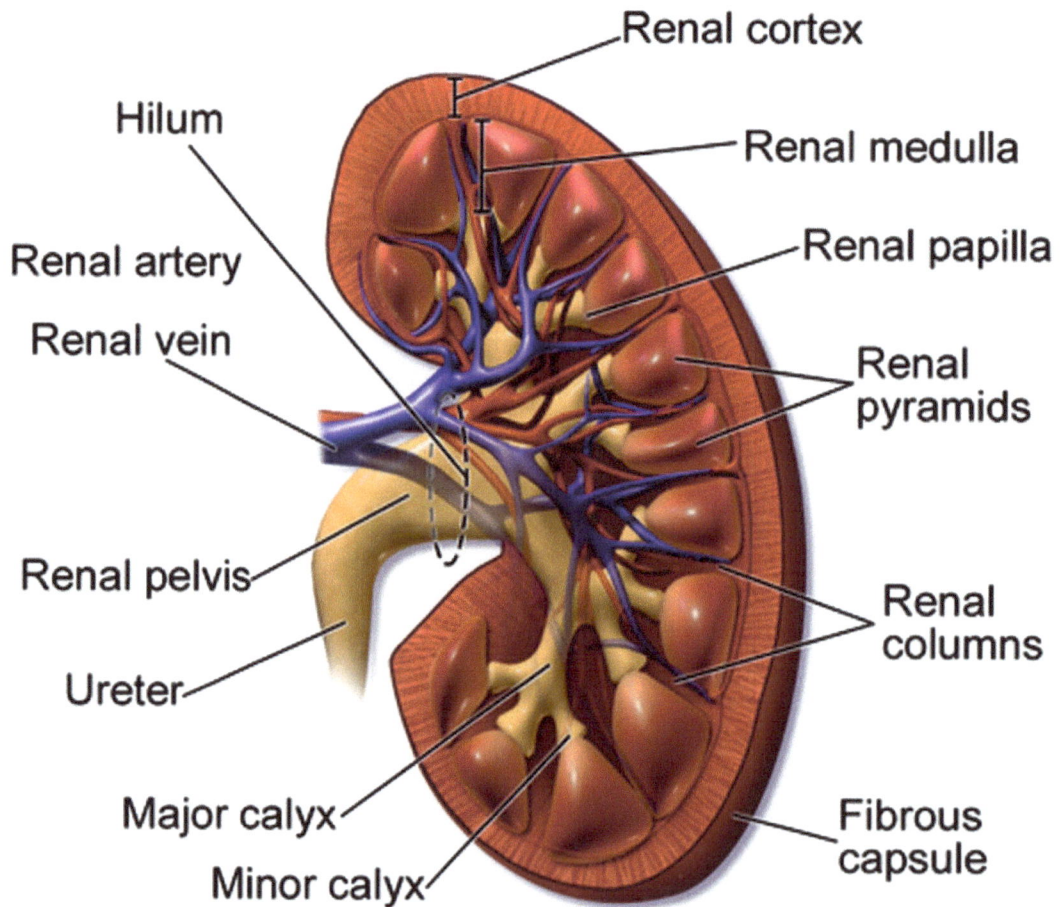

Kidney Anatomy

K is for **Kidneys**. Between you and your heart are the kidneys. Situated on either side of the spine, these two fist-sized organs filter about a half cup of blood every minute, when they're working right. The renal artery carries the blood from the heart into the kidneys, then tiny blood vessels filter it before returning it to the bloodstream through the renal vein. The filtered toxins and waste travel in your urine to your bladder, where it stays until you need to urinate.

Sounds pretty simple, right? Well, it's not. The kidneys balance your electrolytes and minerals, control the pH balance of the blood, make sugar if your blood doesn't have enough, produce hormones that allow you to absorb calcium, and help make red blood cells. The adrenal gland that sits atop each kidney produces cortisol, among other hormones, which helps you deal with stress and a whole lot more.

Some people are born with only one kidney, and some lose one through disease or injury. If you have only one kidney and it starts to fail, you'll need a transplant. Kidney donations have become fairly routine, and the donation often comes from a family member who is a good match. A lot of things can go wrong with your kidneys: various diseases, cancer, cysts, acidosis, azotemia, uremia, total failure—and, of course, kidney stones, which can be caused by any one of those problems. As we age the chance of at least one of these things happening increases. If you smoke, give it up. Cut down on salt. Exercise, drink water, flush out that system, maintain a healthy weight, and watch your blood sugar levels, especially if you have diabetes or want to avoid it. High blood pressure puts you at a high risk of kidney problems.

Urinary tract infections, though common, are less likely if you drink an appropriate amount of water each day, and staying well hydrated also makes you less likely to develop kidney stones. The recommended amount of water to drink daily varies, but about 3 quarts for men and 2 quarts for women seems reasonable. Be careful not to drink too much, though, as overhydration can cause problems too.

Kidney stones can be as small as a grain of sand or as large as a golf ball. You can pass them without even realizing it, or they can cause extreme pain. If one gets trapped in the ureter, the tube from the kidneys to the bladder, it can cause bleeding and keep you from peeing. At that point, surgery might be required. Best to drink plenty of water. Also limit your intake of NSAIDs (nonsteroidal anti-inflammatory drugs) such as aspirin, ibuprofen, and Aleve. They may help with the pain but can have damaging side effects, including ulcers and stomach and heart problems, and they can further adversely affect the kidneys and liver. Keep your kidneys healthy, and they will keep you healthy.

Cool Fact: The kidneys filter about 200 quarts of fluid every day, about enough to fill your bathtub. Some 2 quarts of that fluid, and the waste it carries, are peed out daily; the other 198 quarts are reused within the body.

What other aging problem starts with K?

L

is for
Long Term Care

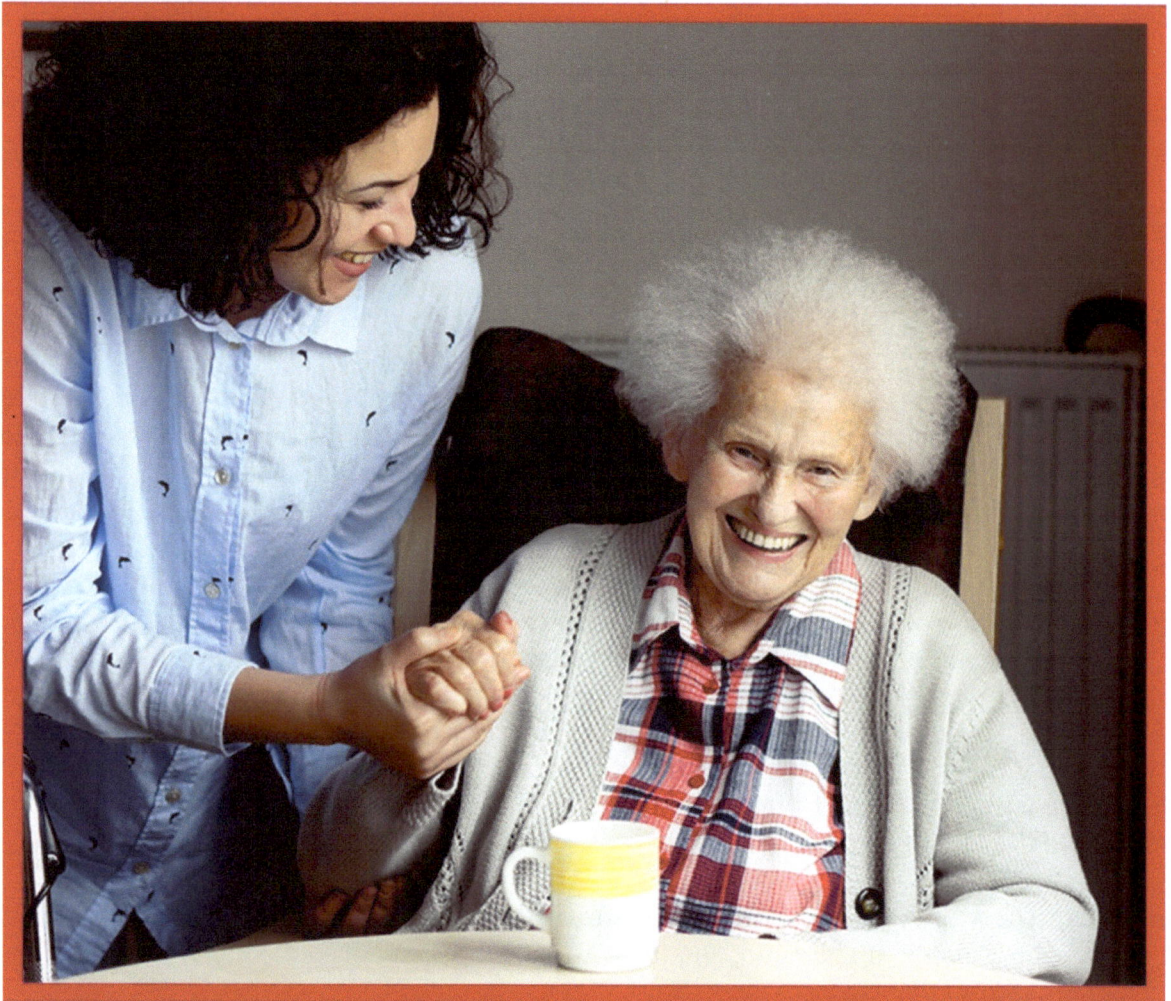

Why don't retirees mind being called seniors?
Because it comes with a 10% discount.
—*Upjokes.com*

L is for **Long-Term Care**. What will you do when you can no longer care for yourself, there are no family members to care for you, you can't afford a full-time live-in assistant, and you need care? The choices are assisted living facilities, nursing homes, and long-term care, either in your own home or in a facility.

Unlike nursing homes, assisted living facilities are not regulated by the federal government, and the definition of "assisted living" varies from state to state. Typically, residents don't require the level of care that is offered by nursing homes, although many assisted living facilities are now accepting those who do need help with all their daily life activities. Accommodations in assisted living can vary from private apartments to shared spaced that resemble dormitories. Facilities built in compliance with the Americans with Disabilities Act of 1990 (ADA) are designed with wider doorways and passages to accommodate wheelchairs and walkers. Sadly, given our capitalist system, it's not surprising that many for-profit facilities care more about their shareholders than their residents. Cases of mismanagement, understaffing, inadequately trained staff, and criminal behavior have been exposed in many such facilities.

Long-term care services are available in your own home if that's what you prefer and can afford. The same services are provided as in assisted living facilities and nursing homes, but usually not 24/7. DADS, the Department of Aging and Disabilities Services, offers programs covering elder care needs, each with its own rules and policies. What kind of service and care you receive will depend on how much money you can pay or the type of insurance you have. Medicaid only pays so much, and after your death the Medicaid Estate Recovery Program will ask for money from your estate, supposing you have any estate left. Long-term care can cost $70,000 a year or more.

Health care providers, surgeons, doctors, nurses, counselors, aides, those who clean up the daily "little accidents": the staff at every level in these elder care facilities work under the very challenging conditions that such tasks impose, and they deserve the thanks of everyone. Not only the gratitude of those receiving care or the relatives of those in care, whose lives are most impacted by their elders' problems, but the thanks of those of us who are lucky enough to go about our lives untroubled by such concerns. People employed in the administration of these facilities are faced every day with making decisions that can mean life or death for millions of our elders. Already overwhelmed in many states, our elder care system will require concerted efforts so that all aging citizens receive the care they need.

Cool Fact: There are over 30,000 assisted living homes in the US. More than half of the residents are over 85 years of age; 71 percent of these residents are women, and 29 percent are men. By 2060 the number of Americans aged 65 and older will more than double, from today's 46 million to some 98 million!

What other aging problems start with L?

M

is for
Muscle Loss

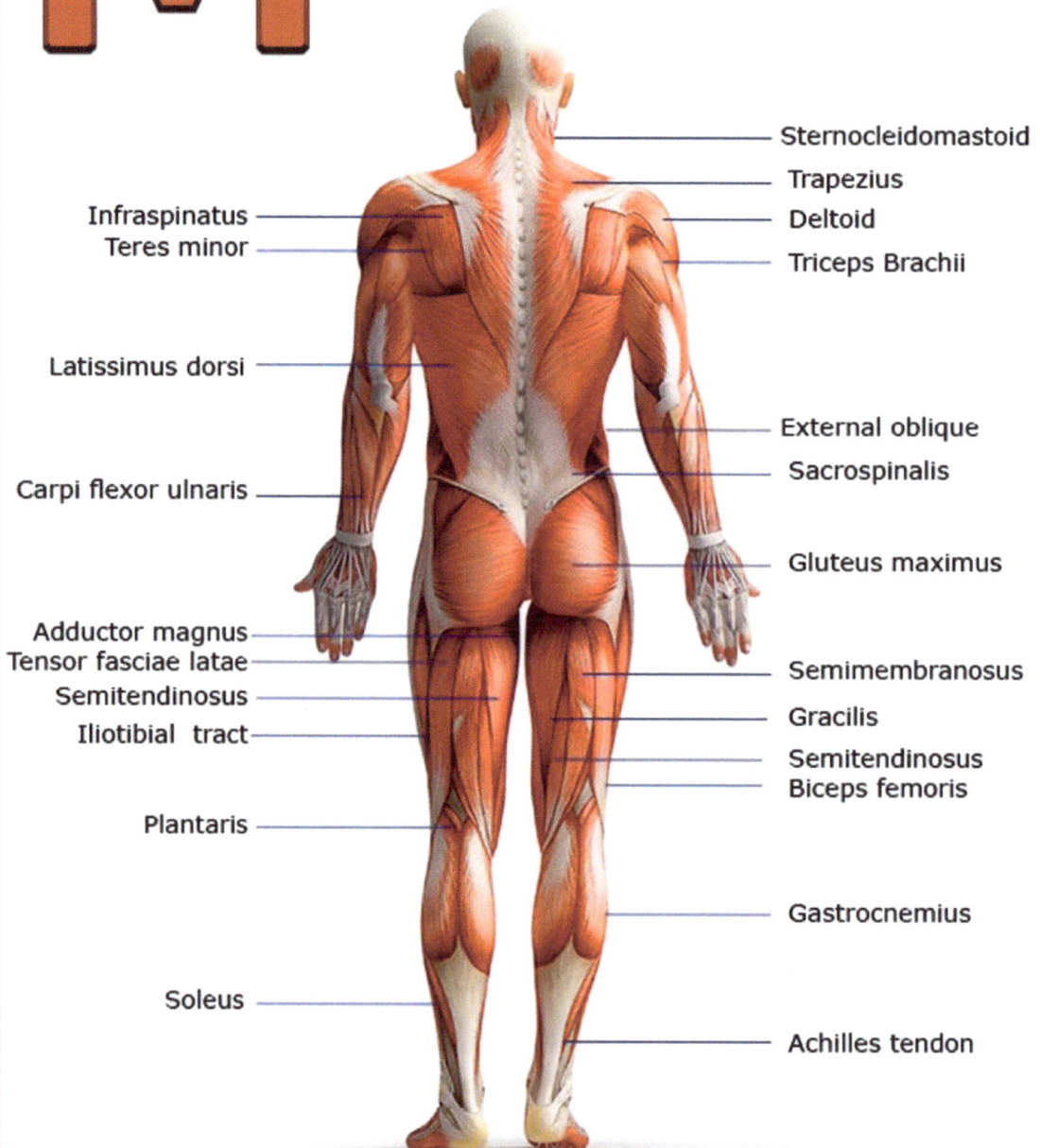

Sternocleidomastoid

Trapezius

Infraspinatus

Deltoid

Teres minor

Triceps Brachii

Latissimus dorsi

External oblique

Sacrospinalis

Carpi flexor ulnaris

Gluteus maximus

Adductor magnus

Tensor fasciae latae

Semimembranosus

Semitendinosus

Gracilis

Iliotibial tract

Semitendinosus

Biceps femoris

Plantaris

Gastrocnemius

Soleus

Achilles tendon

Warning: This page contains strong words: weightlifting, push-ups, biceps, abs, dumbbells, workouts, flexing, sit-ups, pull-ups, bench press.

M is for **Muscle Loss**. The medical term for the gradual loss of muscle mass, strength, and function is *sarcopenia*. Amyotrophy and muscular atrophy are other terms describing a common condition that accompanies aging. Assuming most of us would not look up sarcopenia if we wanted to learn about muscle loss, I've placed it here under M.

Muscle loss, most severe among the sedentary and the frail, is a geriatric problem that can lead to catastrophic decline in the elderly. The gradual loss of muscle strength and function will continue if you don't take action. If you don't act to preserve muscle mass, and if you live long enough, you will likely need full-time care just to survive. Your chance of falls and fractures, which often lead to hospitalization, will increase. If you add obesity to muscle loss, you will be at greater risk of complications. As we have seen with other aging problems, staying physically active and eating a healthy diet will help stave off this unfortunate symptom of the aging process.

As it ages, the body loses its ability to produce hormones and minerals and process the foods we eat, and we have to compensate for these facts. Hormone supplements are being studied, but there are no FDA-approved medications to treat muscle loss as yet. One thing you can do is increase your protein intake, aiming for 2 to 3.5 grams of protein per meal. Including in your diet the vitamins D, C, and E, the dietary supplement creatine, whey protein, other vitamins and minerals, and potassium-rich fruits and vegetables is just as important as exercise. And although it is easier said than done, try to avoid processed foods and to follow the practices outlined elsewhere in this book. Using resistance bands, also recommended for joint therapy, can help you build muscle and melt fat. Sarcopenia can begin as early as your thirties or forties; it accelerates as you reach the age of 65. So the earlier you start taking measures to avoid it, the easier it will be to fight it off. Although aging is the dominant factor in sarcopenia, physical inactivity is the number one contributing factor. Get out and about early in life and keep up your daily activities for as long as you can. The sedentary life only increases muscle loss and other physical effects of aging.

Cool Fact: The Centers for Disease Control and Prevention (CDC) declared sarcopenia a specific disease in 2016. This designation increases the chance of diagnosis and treatment. Not that you will need convincing to address it if you are already—and you likely will be eventually—suffering from muscle loss.

What other aging problems start with M?

N is for Nigerian Prince

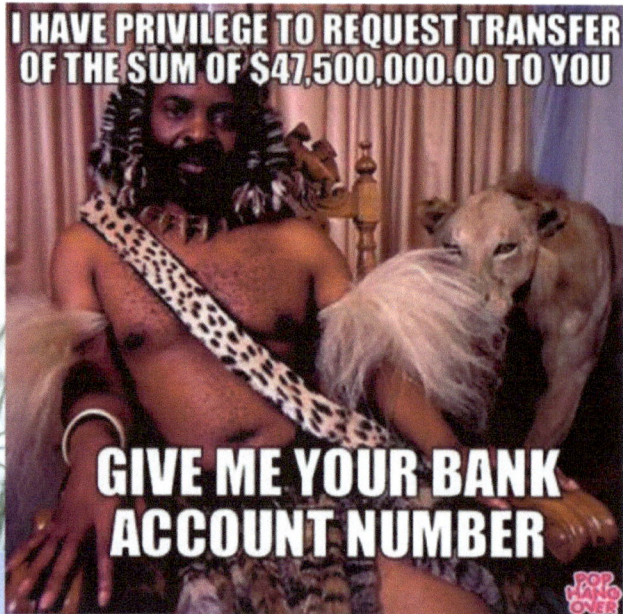
I HAVE PRIVILEGE TO REQUEST TRANSFER OF THE SUM OF $47,500,000.00 TO YOU

GIVE ME YOUR BANK ACCOUNT NUMBER

Dear Sir/Madam,

Blessed birthday greetings from the Nigerian National Petroleum Company. Please kindly provide me with your personal bank account details so that I can transfer you the sum of $40,000,000 as our birthday gift to you.

Yours truly,

Prince Alyusi Islassis

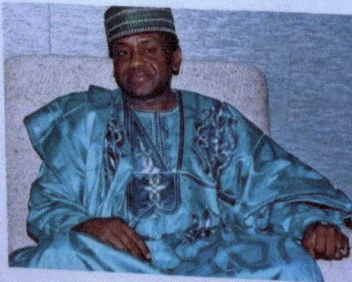

CTV Edmonton @ctvedmonton — Follow

$43M in cash found in empty Nigerian apartment ctvnews.ca/business/43m-i ...

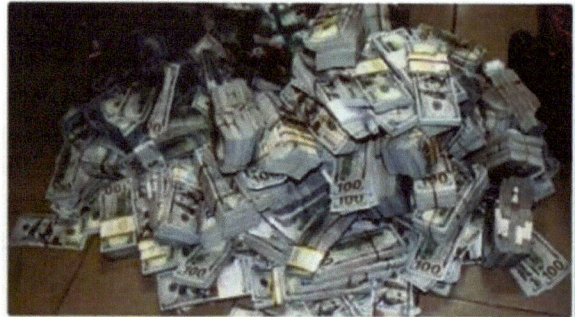

RETWEETS 2,845   LIKES 3,251

Nuck Fuggets @MatHouchens — Follow

Poor guy probably spent the past decade trying to share it but no one ever replied to his email.

N is for **Nigerian Prince.** At some time in your life, you will likely experience what feels like someone jabbing a needle into your foot. That's peripheral neuropathy. It will happen in other parts of your body as well: that's neuropathy. Unpleasant as it is—and it does start with N!—it does not have the devastating and sometimes disastrous effect that falling prey to the Nigerian Prince can have.

The Nigerian Prince scam is a recent version of the 18th-century Spanish Prisoner or Letters for Jerusalem scam, the Black Money scam, and many others. The Nigerian Prince scam—known as the 419 scam, 419 being the section of the Nigerian Criminal Code dealing with fraud—started in the 1980s. Essentially, someone claiming to be a Nigerian prince appeals to you—by phone or on the internet—for help freeing up his millions of dollars by forwarding him a small amount of money. Once he has regained his fortune, he will reward you handsomely for your assistance. Of course, once you have made one investment, other problems arise that require the prince to ask for an additional payment. If you decline, he keeps the payment(s) you've already made, and you never hear from him again. If you do decide to proceed, more things inevitably go wrong. This can continue until you have no money left at all, and then your prince will disappear.

As unlikely as it may sound, many people get sucked in by this appeal, and, not wanting to lose those early payments, they keep doling out more money. Despite widespread publicity about the scam, it continues to circulate. It is estimated that at least $90 million has been raked in so far. Despite raids in Nigeria on rooms full of telephone operators, there are still suites full of operators who may call 500 people or more a day. Even if only 7 percent of those contacted respond, given the thousands of daily calls and emails from thousands of operators, the take quickly adds up.

Such scammers are not only in Nigeria, of course, and scammers have gotten more sophisticated. Originally, the Nigerian Prince would be satisfied with wire transfers of money; now, accessing passwords and personal information is part of a much larger plan. Although millennials report higher rates of fraud, it's still the elderly who, perhaps being more trusting, gullible, naive, or knowing how hard life can be, might feel moved to help—even though they themselves may need additional income. The little old lady and gent, living alone with no one to counsel them, are the most vulnerable and targeted.

Cool Fact: Who said, "You can fool some of the people all of the time and all of the people some of the time, but you can't fool all of the people all of the time"? The quote has been attributed to both Abraham Lincoln and Ainsworth Spofford, the sixth Librarian of Congress, who was appointed by Lincoln. But none of the attributions is verifiable.

What other aging problem starts with N?

O is for Obesity

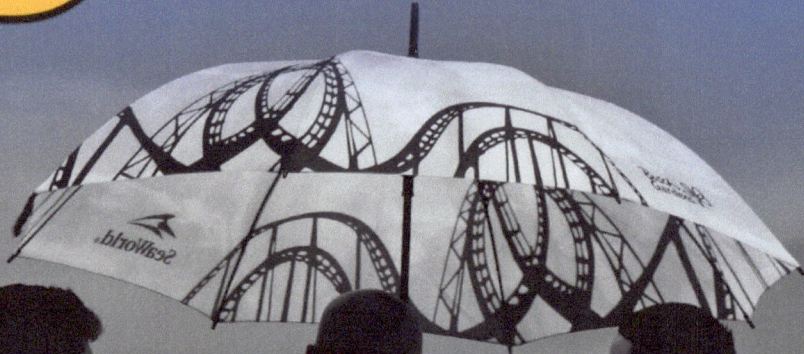

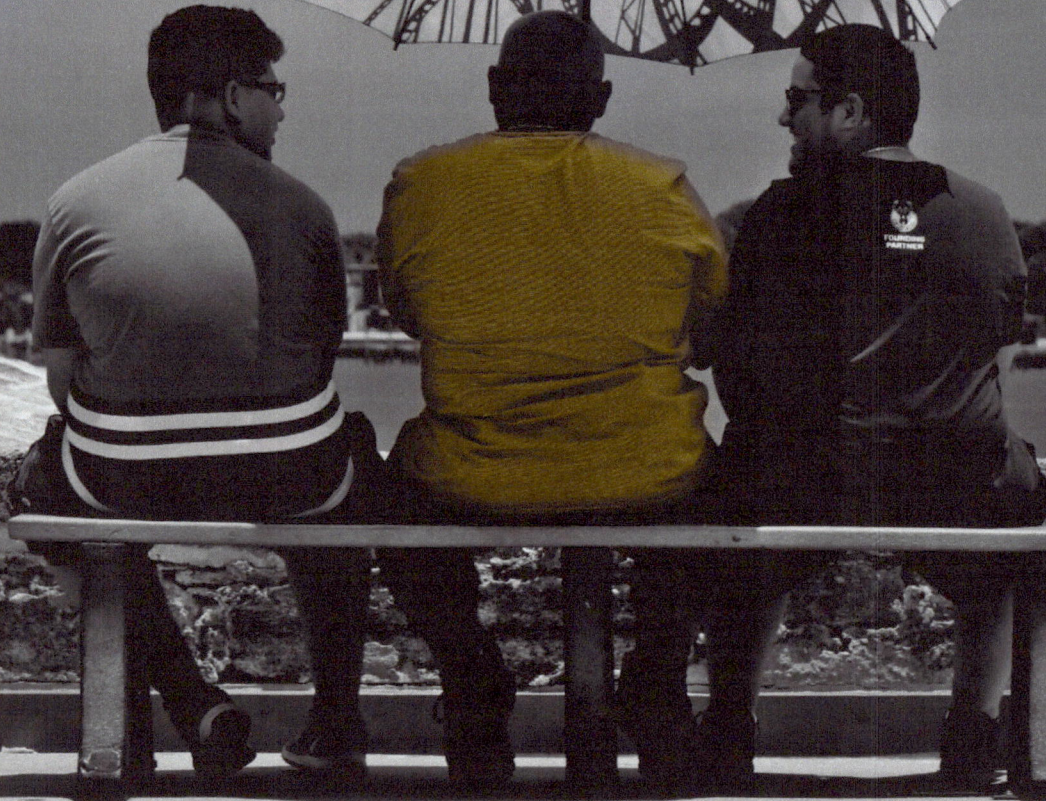

Nutritionist: "You should eat 1200 calories a day."
Fat Guy: "Okay, and how many a night?"

—Jessica Amlee

O is for **Obesity**. Obesity is not a symptom of old age, and the majority of older adults are not obese. But there has been an increase in obesity among all age groups, and the proportion of older adults who are obese has doubled over the past 30 years. Whether you have been obese all your life (80 percent of children born to obese parents will have weight problems) or whether your obesity is due to bad dietary habits, lack of exercise, or decline in the internal functions of the body that occur with aging, it needs to be addressed.

Obesity is a serious, costly, and all-too-common disease. Some of the most common health problems of the aged—arthritis, diabetes, hypertension, and heart disease—are accentuated by obesity. In fact, most of the problems associated with aging are multiplied if you can't get around on your own, and exercise is key to avoiding weight gain. Another perk to exercising: one study found that taking a nap can stave off brain volume loss in the aged, and the more you exercise, the more likely you are to need a nap!

It might help to know what is going on when food comes into the picture. As soon as you see, smell, think about, or taste food, digestive enzymes are released. Once you have eaten, all the digestive operations go into action. But digestion is interfered with by ice-cold drinks, alcohol, and emotional and physical stress, not to mention pesticides, preservatives, pasteurization, overcooking, and lack of fiber. Psyllium fiber curbs the appetite, and we have seen elsewhere that more fiber, fresh vegetables and fruits (particularly fruits like papaya and pineapple), and nuts all improve digestion, and good digestion is essential to avoiding obesity. Soluble fibers absorb 50 times their own weight and make you feel full, helping to prevent overeating and cutting calorie intake.

Obesity is a sign that the body is not getting the HDLs (high-density lipoproteins) it needs. Made by the liver, HDLs carry cholesterol back to the liver for processing and elimination. Inositol is a fat dissolver synthesized by the body from glucose, but empty sugar calories deplete your vitamins and nutrients. Prostaglandins (PG), responsible for 20 percent of total body energy, have low activity in the obese. Refined salt can lead to a sodium deficiency, impairing carbohydrate-to-fat digestion. Magnesium, too, is needed for good digestion. It's a good idea to supplement your CoQ10, DHEA (dehydroepiandrosterone, a steroid hormone), and other vitamins. There are other things that may help: Whey increases gastric juices; kelp boosts the metabolism; prune juice, celery, and cucumber can serve as laxatives. Best to consult a dietician if you need help deciding what to eat.

Cool Fact: The comedian Oliver Hardy was overweight all his life and was known for having a ravenous appetite. After suffering three strokes, Hardy died of cerebral thrombosis at age 65. Stan Laurel was so devastated that he retired and never made another film.

What other aging problem starts with O?

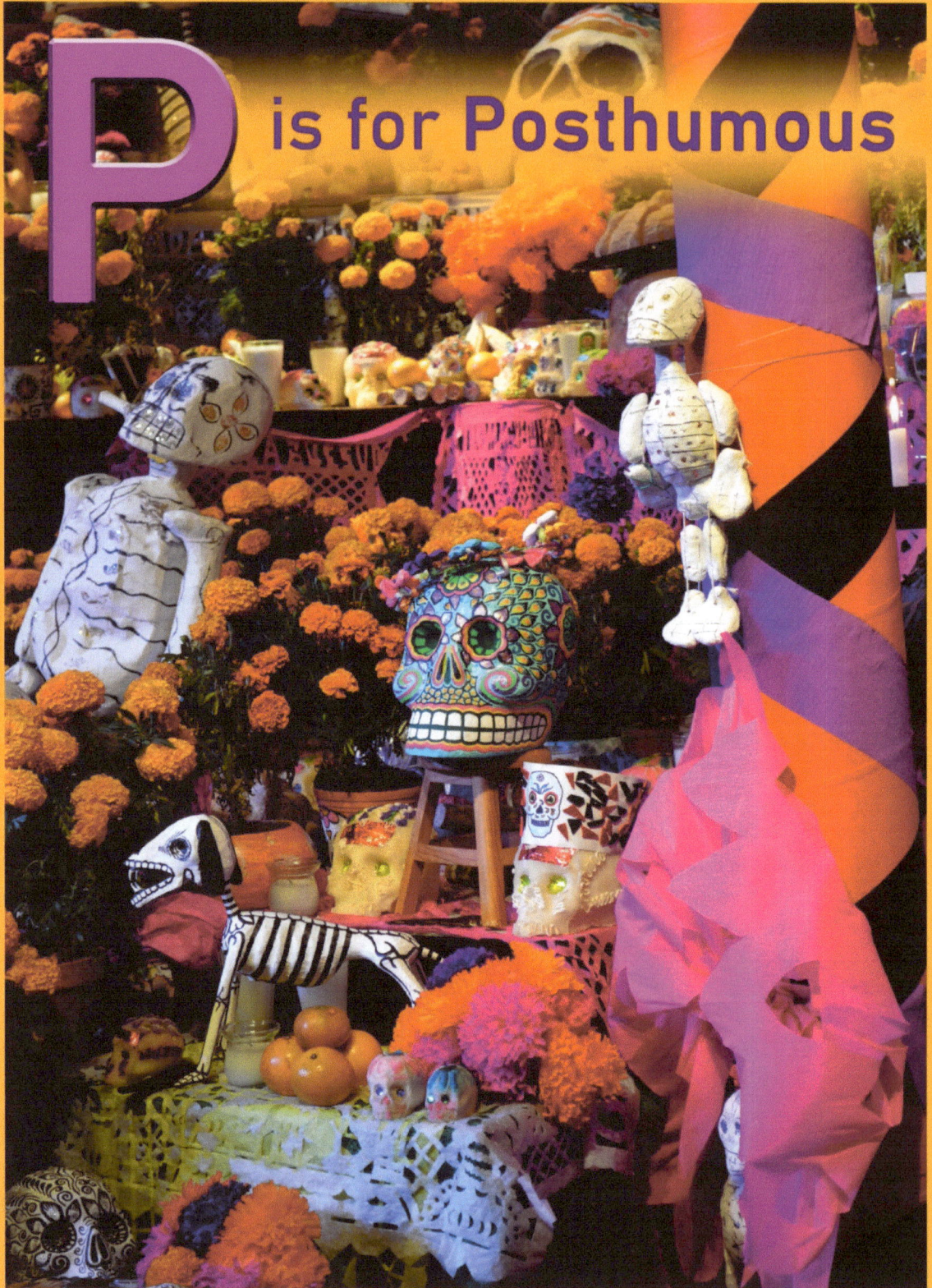

P is for Posthumous

"If you know how quickly people forget the dead, you will stop living to impress people."

—Christopher Walken

P is for **Posthumous**. *Posterus*—Latin for "coming after"—became posthumous, which is a misspelling of posthumus, an alteration of *postumus* ("born after the father's death"). Posthumous recognition for your life's work or accomplishments doesn't do you much good. However, a good deal of energy has been put into praising the dead, often to help those who have "passed over" get benefits that might be available. The *Egyptian Book of the Dead* is perhaps the most comprehensive example of this. The book laid out methods to ensure the best possible afterlife for those who were important or rich enough. Where and when these ideas originated is unknown, but they are assumed to predate the ancient Egyptians. Thousands of years ago, versions of the *Book of the Dead* were inscribed on the walls of chambers and passages in the pyramids and other tombs. The effort to secure unhindered passage to God in the next world, to overcome the opposition of ghostly foes, to endow the entombed body with the power to resist physical corruption, and to ensure a new life in a glorified body in heaven was marked by prayer and elaborate ceremonies. Thereafter, as we see in many other religions, providing the dead with food, drink, and clothing was the duty of surviving family members.

Samsara, the continuous cycle of life, death, and reincarnation, is the basis of Hinduism. The aim of all Hindus is to achieve *moksa*, or salvation, which ends the cycle of rebirth so that one can become part of the absolute soul. One's karma, by which individuals create their own destiny through thought, words, and deeds, can be broken only through surrender to the "eternal truth." In Christianity, after death you are either cremated or stuck in a box and buried. Your soul may go to heaven, where you get a halo, or to hell, where you writhe in eternal fire. In some Islamic versions of heaven, men are surrounded by virgins; it's not clear what women get. In the Indigenous Americas, people who stored their dead above ground (where they could visit and communicate, receiving food and prayers) were criticized by the Catholic Spaniards, who insisted on burial. But Indigenous practices did find their way into Christianity through the institution of el Dia de los Muertos, the Day of the Dead, when families gather at the graves of their departed loved ones for a night of feasting and celebration. Underlying many of these practices is a fear of the dead. Unhappy souls, the walking dead, ghosts, and vampires are thought to roam at night. Different cultures have their own ways of communicating with the dead, and the living regularly call on seers, mediums, clairvoyants, spiritualists, and others who claim psychic powers. Such actions were once considered ecclesiastical offenses punishable by execution, and many a "witch" was convicted for communicating with the dead.

Cool Fact: In 1944 the Scottish medium Helen Duncan was charged and convicted under section 4 of the Witchcraft Act of 1735 for conducting a séance. Duncan appealed the sentence, arguing that she had conjured only friendly spirits that did not fall under the Witchcraft Act, which required that such spirits be wicked or evil.

What other aging problem starts with P?

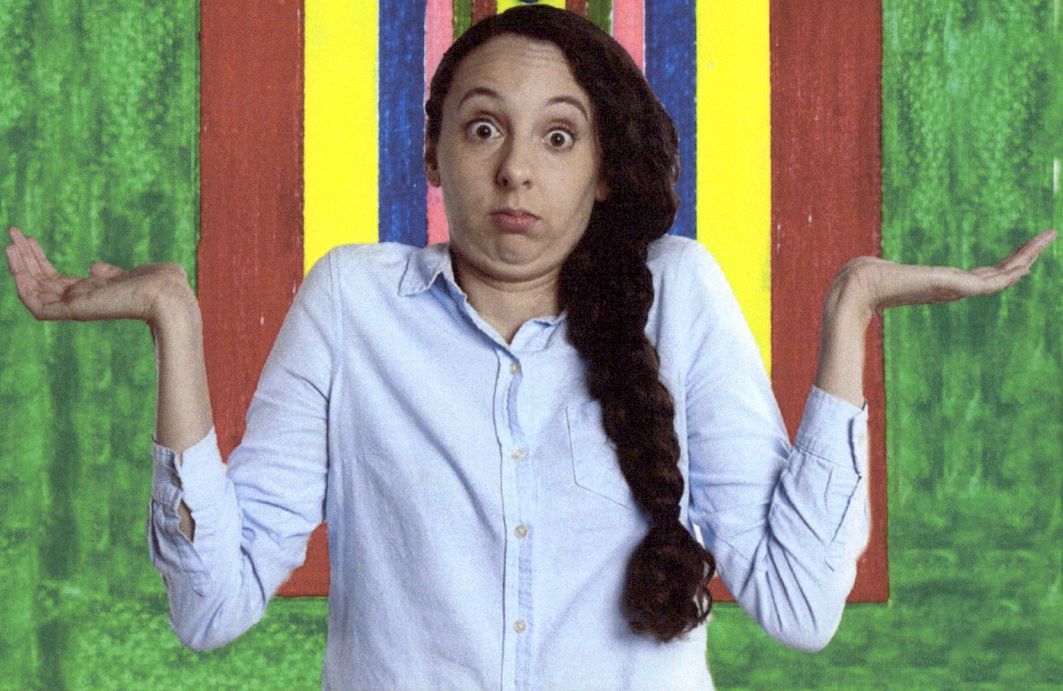

Q is for Question

Q is for **Question.** Aging presents us with questions we didn't have to confront in our younger years. We all have questions; some questions have answers, others don't. Correction: People will give you plenty of answers, but that doesn't mean those answers are valid. They may be comforting, but they may be based on a belief system rather than on facts. Accepting an answer on faith often indicates that there is no definitive answer. Is there a Heaven? Depends on who you ask, what your concept of heaven is, or what version you believe. Questioning accepted ideas is what has kept civilization moving forward and will keep you alert. As we age our brain shrinks, blood flow decreases, and brain plasticity declines, making it harder to learn and remember new things. Any number of things can affect memory: nutritional deficiencies, medications, stress, anxiety, and even hearing loss. And new information can interfere with old memories. All of the bad habits listed elsewhere—heavy drinking, not eating healthy food, avoiding exercise—can impact your memory. Recent studies have found that the edible mushroom known as lion's mane (*Hericium erinaceus*) can improve memory and significantly impact the growth of new brain cells.

Some tips: It's a good idea to write things down, from whether you paid your bills to when you took your medications. If you have close family or friends, confide in them and don't be too proud to ask for help. If you are alone or isolated, reach out. If you are a member of a church, you can usually rely on receiving help there; if you're not a member, you can contact them anyway with your questions and concerns. If you are feeling unwell, I suggest you don't consult your horoscope. Call a doctor instead! She will recommend another professional if she can't figure out what's wrong with you. It may take a while to get a correct diagnosis but keep on asking. If you have chronic physical or mental health problems, you may be able to get disability benefits from Social Security; if you're under 65 you should definitely apply. Once you are on Social Security, applying for disability gets a little more complicated, and you'll have to decide if it's worth the hassle. You may need help with applying, and you'll only find it by asking. Don't call 911 unless you are in an emergency; instead look up city, state, and federal government agencies that offer help through 1-800 numbers or online. You'll find health services, legal services, and social services, including a Department of Aging. Senior Citizen Services offers a wide range of assistance. Find those resources before you need them and keep them close and readily available. Remember that you are not alone.

Cool Fact: Variations of "ask and ye shall receive" appear in each of the books of the apostles in the New Testament, attributing the words to Jesus. In the Old Testament, 1 Kings 3.5, God appears to Solomon in a dream and makes the same offer. Jesus would have known he was quoting God, but his disciples likely did not.

What other aging problem starts with Q?

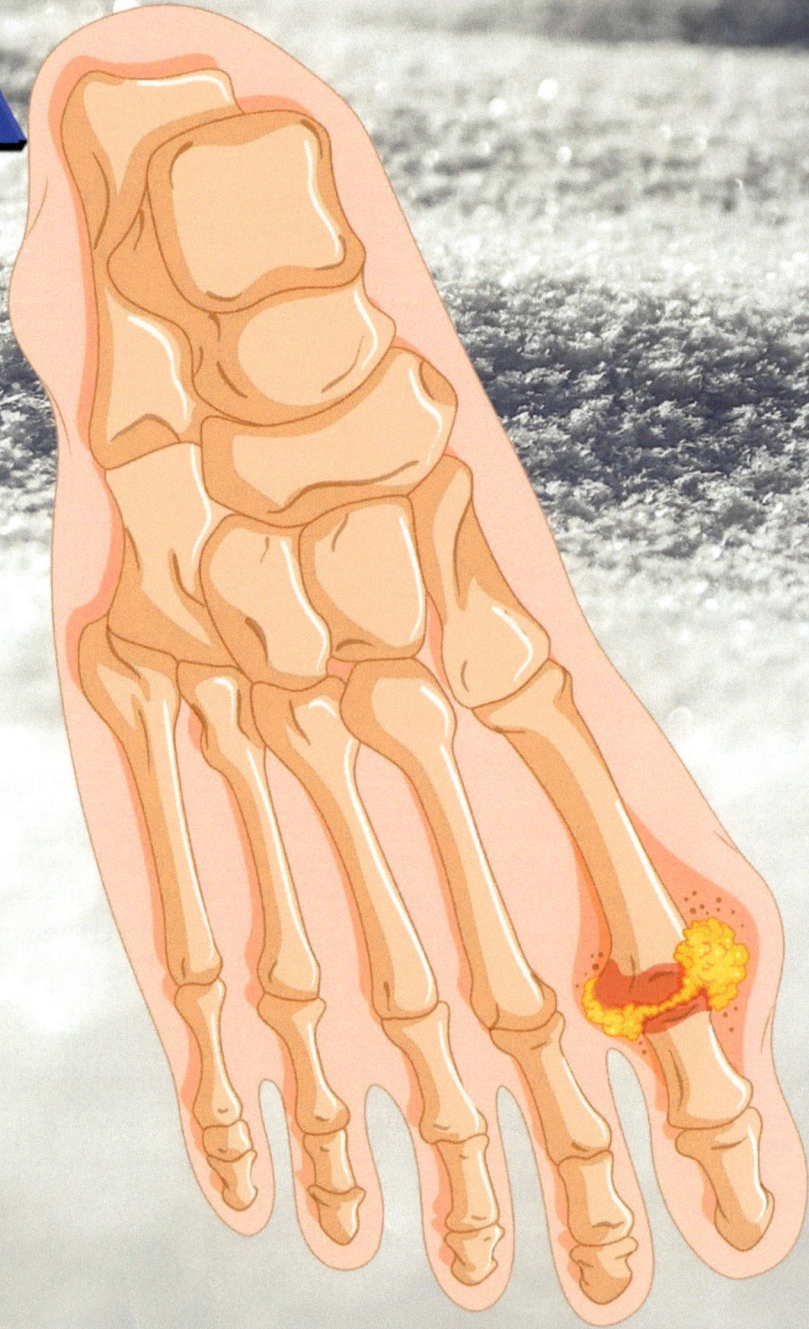

R is for Rheumatism

I have a rheumatism joke, but I can't tell it. It's too inflammatory.

—Acknowledgements to healthgrades.com.

R is for **Rheumatism**. Rheumatism, arthritis—what's the difference? I'm glad you asked. Saying "I have rheumatism" or "I have arthritis" is a simplification. As we saw in *A is for Arthritis*, joint pain is called arthritis. The pain of rheumatism seems to come and go with the weather, and many people say they know the weather is changing because their joints begin to hurt. One reason older people move to Florida is that the warmer climate there helps alleviate their rheumatic symptoms. Just to confuse things, though, we can suffer from rheumatoid arthritis, acute rheumatism, chronic rheumatism, rheumatoid heart disease, rheumatic fever, rheumatism of the loins or muscles (otherwise known as lumbago), polymyalgia rheumatica (which affects twice as many women as men), rheumatism of the thighs (known as sciatica), syphilitic rheumatism, and rheumatic uric acid. In each case, your immune system is attacking healthy body parts. This can be caused by normal "wear and tear" or sustained, repetitive use of that part. Feeling better now? The symptoms are pain or discomfort in the joints, tendons, ligaments, bones, and muscles; stiffness, especially after a period of immobility; and soreness to the touch. Mild exercise helps, but exercise that's too vigorous will worsen your pain. Rheumatism pain can range from relatively minor (a natural part of aging) to disabling or life-threatening. Saunas, hot tubs, warm poultices, massage, acupuncture, topical creams, deep breathing, and meditation help.

Many "natural" substances can relieve pain, and herbs and spices have been employed since antiquity. But unless you are an herbalist, know an herbalist, or are studying to become one, it can be daunting to determine which herbs to take, in what amounts, and in combination with which other herbs; when to gather them, how to store them, and how often to take them. Many herbs have passed the test of time and are not likely to harm you if taken in moderation, but you should always check first with a health professional. Cucumber juice with three parts carrot juice, parsley with celery or carrot juice, black currant tea, Mormon tea, wild chicory root tea, lemon juice, and corn silk tea mixed with dandelion root and golden seal are all said to be good for rheumatism. In fact, the list is endless. Vitamins B6, B15, D3, and E are all important; as with arthritis, calcium helps. Rheumatism can also be treated with hemp. Used for thousands of years as a medicinal, hemp was brought to the Americas in 1611 and became a national crop. In the 1930s, despite the many uses to which hemp was then being put, Harry Anslinger, the first commissioner of the Federal Bureau of Narcotics, decided to criminalize it. (Criminalizing alcohol hadn't worked, I guess they needed to try something else.)

Cool Fact: Copper is an essential nutrient for the body. For centuries people have worn copper bracelets to reduce the pain or inflammation of rheumatic arthritis. Medical studies have found no cause-and-effect connection between the two, but since pain can flare up and then subside, if one is wearing a copper bracelet it would be easy to link the two. Whether it is the "placebo effect" or not, if it works for you, why not use it? (Fish oil is better. Avoid aluminum.)

What other aging problems starts with R?

S is for Senility

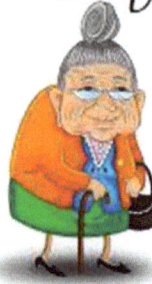

The Senility Prayer

Grant me the senility to forget the people I never liked anyway, the good fortune to run into the ones I do, and the eyesight to tel. the difference.

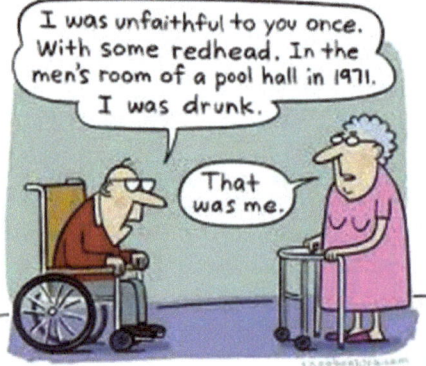

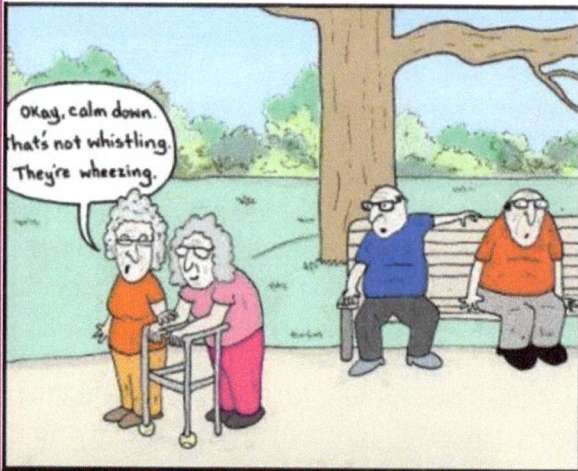

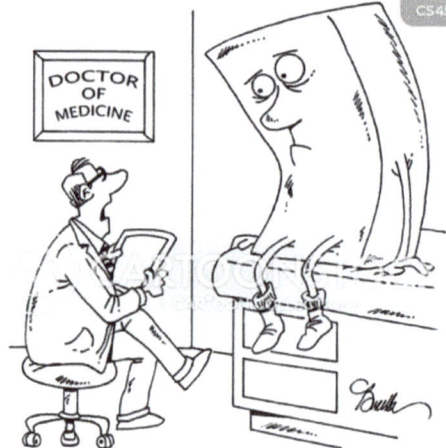

"Nothing to be concerned about. Short-term memory foam loss is very common in a mattress your age."

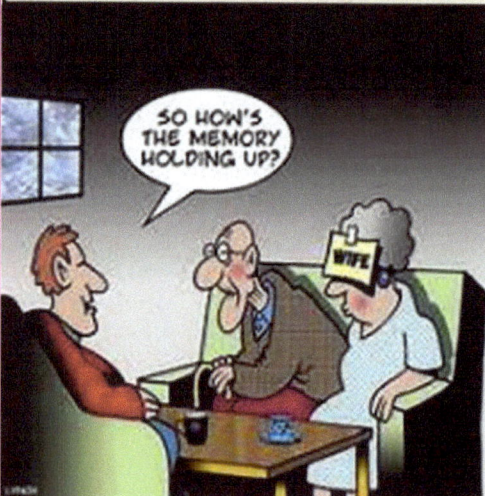

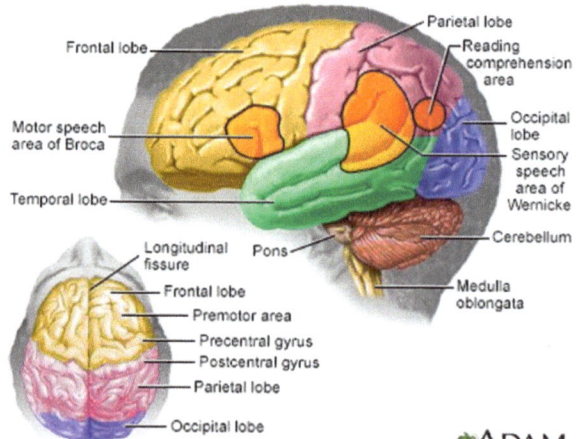

A nursing home attendant says to an old resident, "I think it's so nice
that you still call your wife darling, honey, and love."
The old man replies, "Well, I've forgotten her name and I'm afraid to ask her."

—Senior Citizen Jokes.htm

S is for **Senility**. You may laugh, but senility, or senile dementia, isn't funny. According to a 2013 Alzheimer's Association report, 1 in 3 adults over the age of 65 dies with dementia or Alzheimer's, sometimes because dementia led to respiratory failure. Doctors don't use the terms "senility" or "senile" these days; "neurocognitive disorder" is preferred to describe different types of dementia. Even though the medical community no longer employs the term, we all know what it means when someone becomes "senile." And while "senility" may be used to refer to dementia, "dementia" is not necessarily linked to aging; it is an umbrella term for Alzheimer's disease, Lewy body dementia, vascular dementia, frontotemporal dementia, Parkinson's disease, and Huntington's disease. Although most cases of dementia occur in people over 65, younger people can develop it as well.

Confused? Well, that doesn't mean you have dementia or are going senile. But getting lost in a familiar neighborhood, using the wrong word to refer to a known object, forgetting names of family members or friends, forgetting things that happened in the past, or needing help finishing tasks that never used to be a problem can be signs of dementia. Many conditions that can lead to intellectual impairment are reversible, including conditions like hypothermia, hypoglycemia, vitamin deficiency, and long-term alcohol abuse. Properly treated, your symptoms will lessen if you address these issues, so check with a physician.

Actual senile dementia is caused by irreplaceable brain cells wasting away due to narrowing and hardening of the arteries that carry blood to the brain, supplying it with oxygen and nutriments. Little can be done to stop its progress. Considering the pollution, we are all exposed to and the toxins in the food we eat, it may not be surprising that dementia is so prevalent. What can we do to prevent ourselves from suffering the effects of "neurocognitive disorder"? Start early. As with everything else, living a healthy life, staying physically and mentally active, avoiding stress, eating a healthy diet, and protecting yourself from occupational and environmental risks will help. Having a positive and optimistic attitude can improve the quality of your life and chances of longevity. There are also prescription medications and other treatments that can improve brain function, and various teas, herbs, and vitamins can help alleviate those occasional "senior moments."

Cool Fact: In 1906, German psychiatrist and neurologist Alois Alzheimer performed an autopsy on a woman who had died after suffering memory loss and other symptoms of dementia. He found misshapen clumps of protein and twisted bundles of fiber in her brain, as well as shrinkage around the nerve cells. In 1910, Emil Kraepelin, who worked with Alzheimer, codified his colleague's findings and named the condition "Alzheimer's disease."

What other aging problem begins with S?

T is for Tinnitus

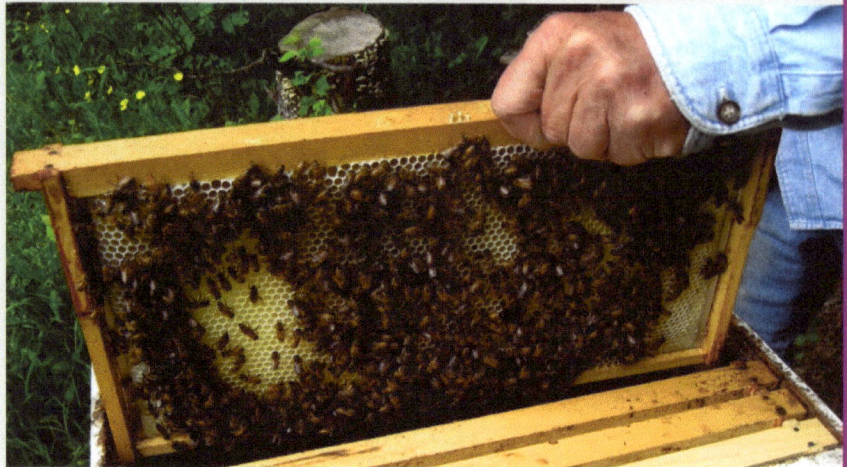

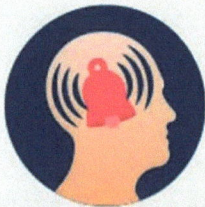

TINNITUS

Tinnitus is the perception of noise or ringing in the ears. A common cause of tinnitus is inner ear hair cell damage.

SYMPTOMS

- Ringing
- Buzzing
- Roaring
- Clicking
- Hissing
- Humming

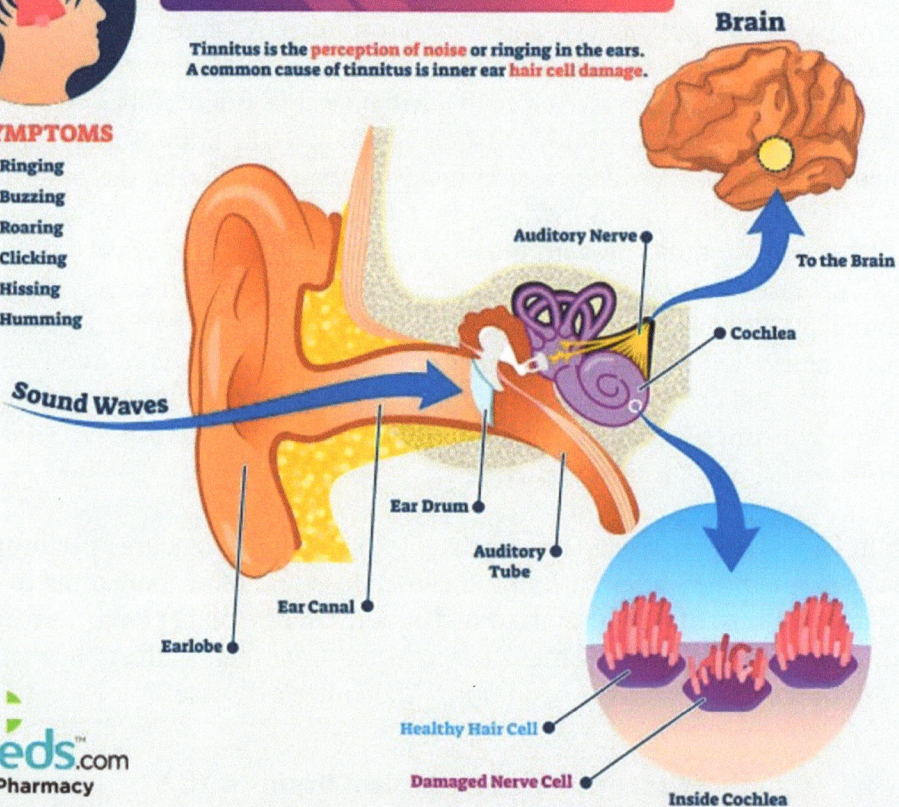

Brain

To the Brain

Auditory Nerve

Cochlea

Sound Waves

Ear Drum

Auditory Tube

Ear Canal

Earlobe

Healthy Hair Cell

Damaged Nerve Cell

Inside Cochlea

netmeds.com
India Ki Pharmacy

That tinny ringing in your ears? Yes, it's tinny tus. It's the same as tin I tus, and just as annoying.

—M.E.

T is for **Tinnitus**. Ringing, buzzing, hissing, roaring, whistling, or a combination of all of these: that's tinnitus. Though it's a common problem for the elderly, it can start when you are young, and certainly the damage starts early on and increases with time. Someone should have warned you when you were young or provided you with ear protectors. Chainsaws, buzz saws, motorcycles, leaf-blowers, blow dryers, the hand dryers found in public toilets, loud music blasting out of that speaker you were standing next to at a rock concert, fireworks, firing a gun (especially a shotgun), even the garbage disposal or vacuuming—all can damage the delicate hair cells or sensitive nerves in your ears.

Any noise above 75 decibels should be avoided, especially by children. All of the noises listed above register over 100 decibels; the shotgun is 140 decibels. Few target shooters and very few hunters wear ear protection; the longer they hunt, the more likely tinnitus and hearing loss will result. An estimated 50 million Americans are afflicted. So what can you do? Not a lot. Founded in 1971, the American Tinnitus Association (ATA) has been providing grants for tinnitus research, support groups that offer coping strategies, and information to help those who are so badly affected that they can't sleep, are stressed and tense, or driven to distraction. So far, no cure has been found.

Supplements are advertised that may offer some relief; these contain ingredients that have proved to improve circulation to the ear and prevent fat deposits from forming in them. Some help, but others are worthless. Google Consumer Review for their suggestions. The ATA says that caffeine, alcohol, nicotine, high-sugar foods, tonic water, and certain medications can make tinnitus worse, as can stress and fatigue. If you have hearing loss in addition to tinnitus, wearing hearing aids can help decrease the volume of tinnitus relative to the sounds of everyday life that you were not hearing so well before. Distractions of any kind can take your mind off the sound, and playing soft music can bring relief. Whenever you concentrate on something, whether it's work, exercise, yoga, or meditation, the focus required takes your mind off the tinnitus, if only temporarily. Joseph Marion states that tinnitus can be caused by wax buildup, ear infection, or sodium potassium imbalance. He suggests taking vitamin B3, Ginko biloba, fenugreek seed tea, and black cohosh, or even putting onion juice drops in the ears. Thyroid disorders as well as some medications, prescription or over-the-counter, could contribute to tinnitus. Given that such a wide variety of things can be responsible for the problem, use caution and consult with a physician before treating it—as always!

Cool Fact: If tinnitus is bringing you down, it's time to take a mental health day. Turn off the computer, go for a walk, exercise, or get into something that demands all of your attention— something that's relaxing, fulfilling, and makes you happy.

What other aging problem starts with T?

U is for Urination

HELLO, YOU'VE REACHED THE INCONTINENCE HOTLINE.

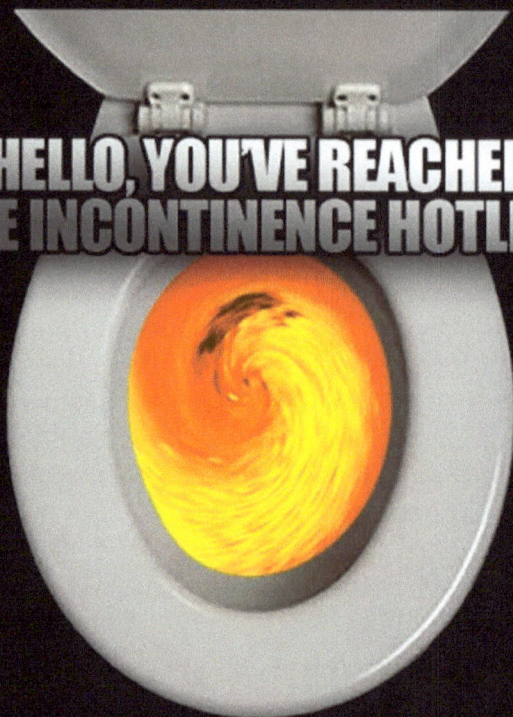

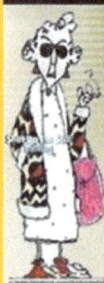

CAN YOU PLEASE HOLD?

PainfulPuns.com

You know you're gettin' OLD when you can't walk past a bathroom without thinking "I may as well pee while I'm here."

Minnie Pauz....

©dAdams www.minniepauz.com

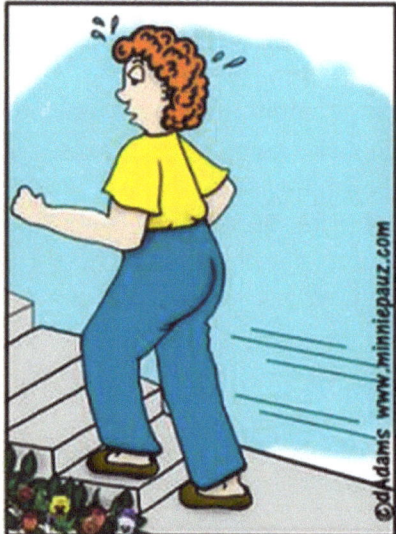

How am I supposed to take a 2 mile walk when I can't go two feet without having to go to the bathroom?

If my body were a car I would trade it in on a newer model.. Everytime I cough sneeze or sputter my radiator leaks and my exhaust backfires..

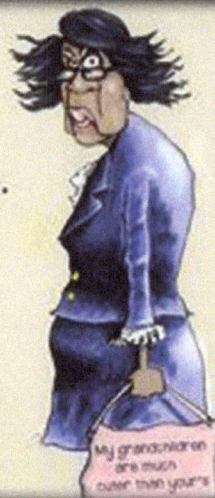

*Two elderly couples are talking, one wife hears her husband tell the other
that when he has to get up in the night to pee, the good Lord turns the light on for him.
"Oh, no." She says to her friend. "He's peeing in the refrigerator again."*

U is for **Urination**. There are many urinary problems, and they increase as we age. Incontinence is the most common, affecting males and females alike. "Having to go" can be problematic under many circumstances. You may not have to make your way to the outhouse anymore, but staggering to the bathroom several times a night, as most elderly folks must do, can be fraught with dangers—especially if you had a glass of wine or two. Falls cause 40,000 deaths per year in the elderly and countless nonfatal breaks and bruises. Also, having to get up to use the bathroom disrupts one's sleep, and it can be difficult to get back to sleep. To avoid this you can keep a jug by the side of the bed: when you awaken, just reach over, grab the receptacle, relieve yourself, carefully return it to the floor, and be back to sleep in no time. Women can use a "pStyle" device, standing or squatting.

Incontinence, though inconvenient, is the least of the urinary problems we can face. An enlarged prostrate is the most common cause of frequent urination in men, but the issue could be a urinary tract infection that can progress to a serious kidney infection. Cystitis, or bladder infection, affects more women than men; if vaginitis is the problem, discharge in various colors may be accompanied by cramps and back pain. Prostatitis advances as we age, making "going" an urgent need that, if ignored or delayed, will lead to embarrassing leaks.

The water you drink—whether it's soft or hard, the amount, its source, and the way it is conveyed—can also affect your system. According to Joseph Marion, over 2,100 chemicals are in American water supplies; 156 are carcinogens; and 26 of those can spur tumor growth. A possible result: bladder cancer. The kidneys filter harmful chemicals from the body via the bladder, and the chemicals you have been exposed to in your work or living habits, smoking, and certain foods increase your risk for bladder issues as you age. As with every other health problem, there are plenty of alleged quick fixes out there. Your doctor may know which, if any, are useful. Some plants have proven effective: juniper (which acts as a diuretic), winter cherry, marshmallow, mugwort, nettle, horsetail, and knotweed, to name a few. Cranberry, both the juice and the berries, contains chemicals that prevent disease-causing bacteria from attaching to the walls of the urinary tract. How and whether you should try such remedies is for your medical specialist to answer.

*As we were about to leave, I said to my French friend,
"Do you need to use the bathroom?" He said, "oui oui." —M.E.*

Cool Fact: Before the invention of indoor plumbing, the chamber pot was used by one and all. Cabinets to house the pots were often finely made pieces of furniture. King Henry VII's "groom of the stool" (the closed stool or night commode, also called the necessary stool, night stool, or night commode), whose official title was The Groom of the King's Closed Stool, was the highest ranked among those who attended to the king's personal needs. Elizabeth I had a Lady of the Chamber for the same purpose.

What other aging problem starts with U?

V is for Vertigo

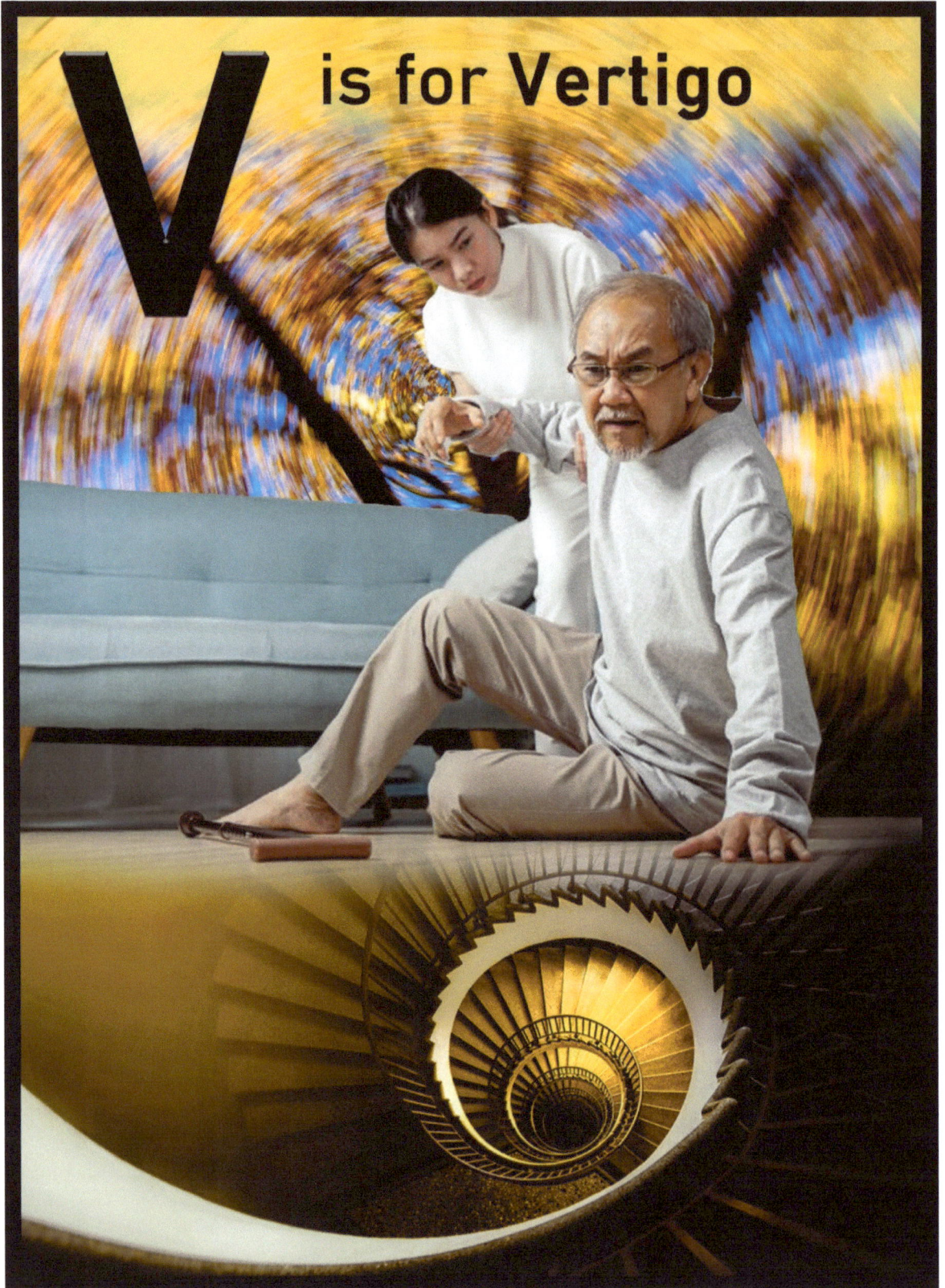

The world does not revolve around you.

You're just dizzy.

V is for **Vertigo**. Vertigo, dizziness, and loss of equilibrium that often affect the elderly can be due to a number of ailments. Inner ear injury, irregular blood pressure, motion sickness, Meniere's syndrome, multiple sclerosis, or a low blood oxygen condition may be contributing factors. These days, a high ozone level in cities is considered dangerous; at the beach or in the mountains, it's considered healthful. Sodium (not to be confused with salt) is an essential mineral, but excess levels cause many problems, while sodium deficiency leads to dizziness and vertigo. Anemia, parasites in the body, teeth clenching or grinding, dairy allergy, even Valium—and of course, spinning around too fast—can cause vertigo. But vertigo is no joke, and if you're experiencing dizziness, lie down before you fall down.

Most often vertigo is related to damaged organs of balance in the inner ears. As noted elsewhere, our hearing is under attack most of our lives, so it's not surprising that the elderly in particular suffer from poorly functioning ears. Labyrinthitis, an infection usually caused by a virus that disrupts the ear's fluid-filled chambers that control balance, results in extreme vertigo. It is not a dangerous condition and goes away when the virus clears up. Meniere's disease comes about from an increase of fluid in the labyrinth of the inner ear, exerting pressure that disturbs one's sense of balance. Generally, the disorder is mild and clears up on its own, but a bad case can cause deafness. Consult an ear, nose, and throat (ENT) specialist if your symptoms persist. The symptoms of multiple sclerosis (MS), a chronic disease of the central nervous system, include dizziness and balance problems that can vary from day to day. A physiotherapist can offer simple exercises to manage these issues—exercises that will help anyone with vertigo. Good posture and suppleness, things we tend to lose with age, can benefit your balance. Tai chi, outdoor walking, and other exercise will help. Joseph Marion recommends vitamins B2, B3 (Niacin), B12, and folic acid along with the herbs feverfew, Gingko biloba, lemon balm, lily of the valley, linden, mistletoe, stinging nettle, rosemary, and thyme (but not parsley and sage). An herbalist may know what form and amounts these herbs may be taken in—but don't ever experiment on yourself.

Cool Fact: In Alfred Hitchcock's 1958 film *Vertigo*, the character played by James Stewart has a pathological fear of heights. A woman he has been paid to follow ascends a tower and falls to her death (or seems to)—due in part to the crippling fear of heights? Later, Stewart's character meets a woman who closely resembles the "dead" woman. She is in fact, the same person and (spoiler alert!) falls to her death from the tower again. (It's an elaborate murder plot.) But Hitchcock got it wrong: the fear of heights is acrophobia, not vertigo!

What other aging problems start with V?

W is for Will

Wills of the

RICH

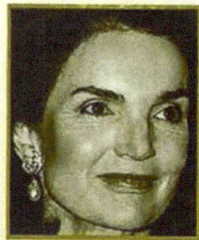 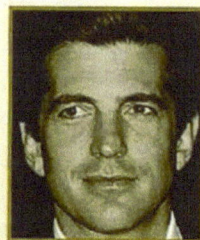

& FAMOUS

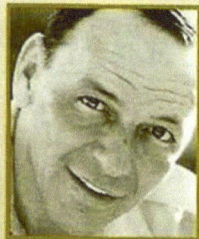 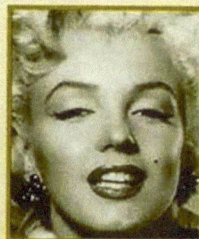 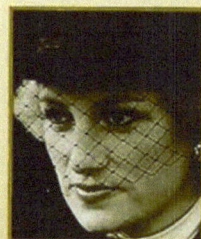

A Fascinating Glimpse at the Legacies of Celebrities

Herbert E. Nass, Esq.

Death is not the end.
There remains the litigation over the estate.

—*Ambrose Bierce*

W is for **Will**. Your will: Get it written! Procrastination is not a good move in this case. Too many people say "I'll get to it later"—and then they up and die. We all leave something behind when we die, even if it's only debts, so if you have family, putting instructions in a will can make it easier for them to deal with your "estate." Depending on how big, diverse, varied, or complicated your estate is, getting the assistance of an estate lawyer—or any lawyer who writes up wills—is worth the cost. If you're not leaving much behind, you can go online and find a form that will allow you to prepare a will.

You also need to let those you leave behind know what you want to have done with your body. If there is a family plot in a cemetery or if you have bought a plot, then there will be the cost of getting your body to the site and into the ground. Hopefully, you'll leave money for that expense. Cremation, while it's not so good for the atmosphere, at least means that a piece of land won't be rendered useless forever. Your loved ones will have to decide what to do with your ashes unless you spell it out for them. Water cremation is becoming a popular alternative, and it's a more environmentally friendly method than dispersal in the air. Natural organic reduction (human composting) is another method being explored. Alternatively, you might donate healthy body parts to those in need or give your entire body to science. Registerme.org and organdonor.gov are two sites that can help with that. In the U.S., 16 people die every day waiting for a donor organ.

The more specific you are in your will, the less chance there is of litigation and arguments over who is going to get what. Homes, land, property, and rights of all kinds can be lost when there is no will. Shortly after the Osage tribe was forced to move to Oklahoma, oil was discovered there, and many members of the Osage Nation became very rich. This led to the "Reign of Terror" after white opportunists learned that they could automatically inherit the oil rights of an Osage wife. Hundreds of unsolved murders of Osage owners of oil rights occurred as white husbands poisoned or otherwise disposed of their Osage wives and even children who would have legally inherited the rights. Inheritance laws vary from state to state but dying without a valid will ("intestate") can only complicate matters for your survivors. If you don't spell it out, they will have to fight it out. If you don't seek good advice or a good lawyer, those you leave behind will need to do just that. Fortunes may be lost for the want of a well-thought-out will.

Cool Fact: The wealthy Portuguese noble Luis Carlos de Noronha Cabral de Camara had no offspring and few friends. He chose 70 names at random from a phone book and split his fortune between them. In 2007 they received around 7,000 euros each.

What other aging problem starts with W?

X is for X-Ray

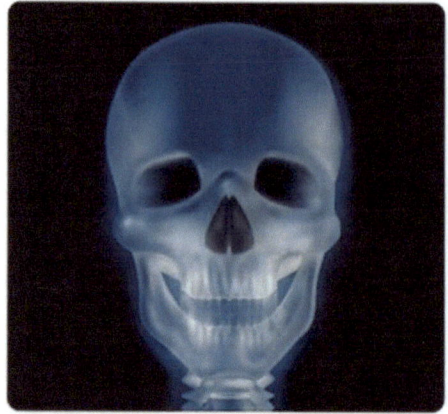
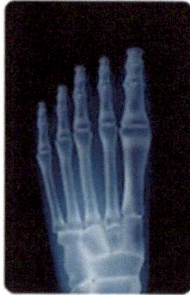
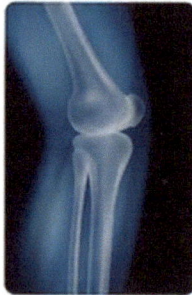
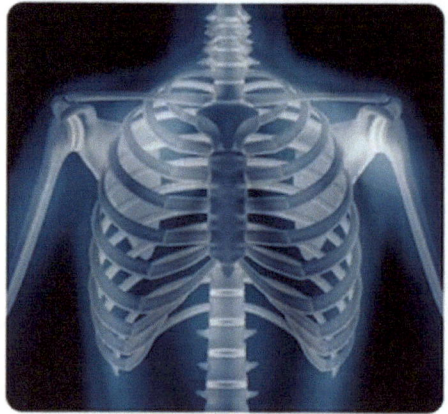
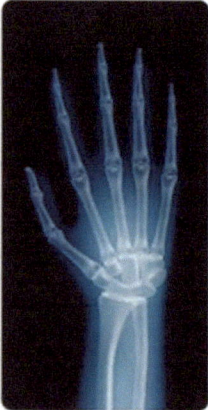
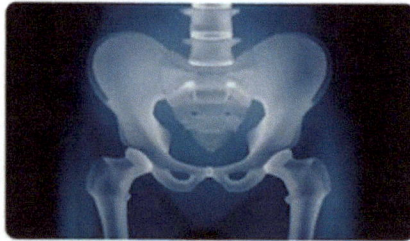
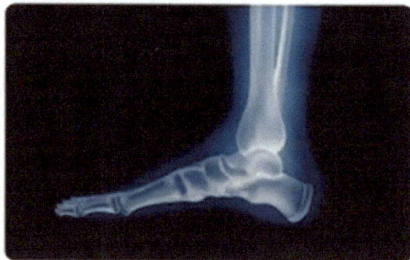
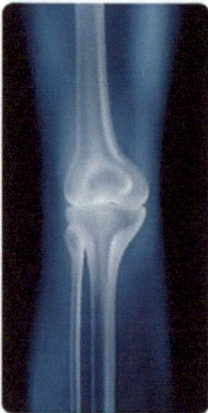
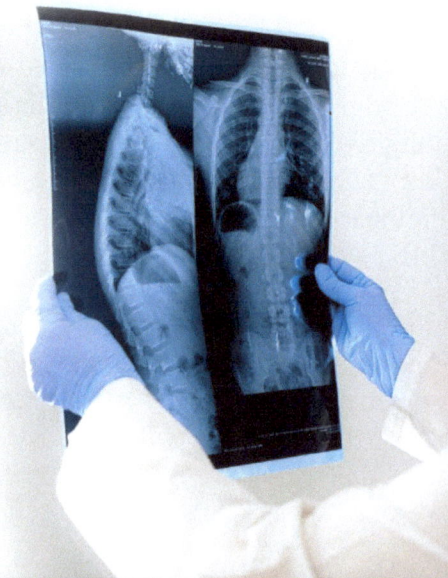

X is for **X-Ray.** W. C. Röntgen (1845–1923), while experimenting with cathode rays, found new rays he called X-rays. His work won him the Nobel Prize in physics. X-rays allow for non-invasive examination of medical issues and monitoring of a treatment's progress. They help guide the insertion of catheters, stents, and other devices into the body. They aid in the removal of blood clots and other similar blockages. An X-ray may reveal problems like bone infections, tumors, and gas or fluid in areas where there should be none. Radiology, the most familiar kind of X-ray, is used to look at broken bones, teeth, and the chest, and it uses the least amount of radiation. Fluoroscopy, in which the patient lies on a table that passes through a ring-shaped scanner, is a kind of X-ray that can watch activity in the body; it uses a little more radiation than radiology or a CT (computed tomography) scan. As the body moves through the scanner, a series of images are made to build up a 3D image, using the highest dosage of scanning radiation. A CT scan of the abdomen delivers the equivalent of 2.7 years of natural background radiation, which is the amount we are exposed to going about our normal daily lives. Airplane fliers and astronauts are exposed to higher doses of cosmic radiation at higher altitudes.

X-rays are classed as carcinogens. It is estimated that there were at least 62 million CT examinations performed in the U.S. during 2007 that could result in 29,000 future cancers, based on current risk estimates. But a recent study questioned whether very low X-ray exposure can cause cancer, claiming that whatever damage it might cause is repaired by the body. The threshold for permanent damage is thought to be far higher than standard X-ray doses from any kind of scan. This only applies to adults, however; children are at greater risk. There is no doubt that in contributing to the right diagnoses and courses of treatment, X-rays are more beneficial than dangerous. Still, I wouldn't refuse that heavy lead blanket being placed on your chest when having your teeth X-rayed at the dentist.

Cool Fact: X-rays allow scientists to investigate the insides of Egyptian mummies that are thousands of years old without having to open them up and take them apart. They can also see the artifacts buried along with them. One mummy of a child was found to have a small piece of calcium carbonate in the shape of a scarab beetle embedded in its abdomen. The scarab is the ancient Egyptian symbol of rebirth and of the soul.

What other aging problem starts with X?

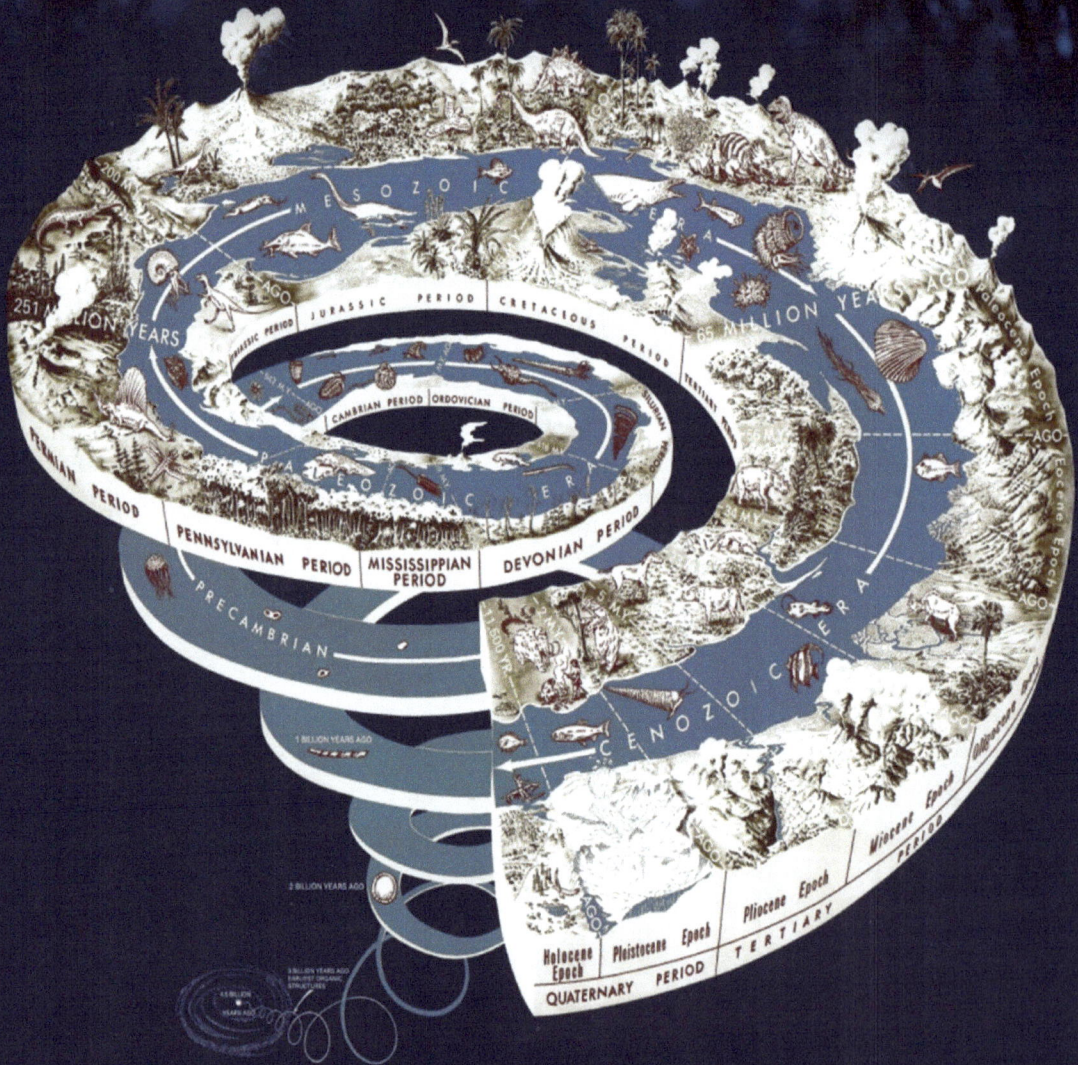

Y is for Years

> "You don't stop laughing when you get old,
> you get old when you stop laughing."
>
> —*George Bernard Shaw*

Y is for **Years**. "Four score and seven years." If you are 87, as the nation was when Abraham Lincoln made his speech, you have lived longer than most of your peers. In the U.S., the average life expectancy fell in 2021, and the country now has the lowest life expectancy rate among large wealthy nations: 73.5 years for males, 79.3 years for females. Japan has the highest at 81.5 for males, 87.6 for females. The gap between men and women has widened more in the U.S. than in other comparable nations, partly due to the cost of healthcare. Even though America outspends its peers in wealthy countries on healthcare, it still has the lowest life expectancy. Japan, with the lowest per-person health spending worldwide, maintains the highest life expectancy.

As the years go by, taking care of your health becomes ever more important. Throughout this book, we have looked at various ways in which the elderly can maintain or improve their health. Of course, there are individuals who drink, smoke, eat badly, don't exercise, and yet live on while family and friends bite the dust. But those are the exceptions! There is no doubt that having a good, healthy regimen pays off. Generally, wives in the U.S. are younger than their husbands, and since women usually live longer than men, half of the widows over the age of 65 outlive their spouses by 15 years. There are 11.8 million widows in the U.S., with 2,800 added every day. Those years after a husband's death can be very challenging, as many widows don't have a savings plan and are faced with financial burdens once shared with their husband. In addition, they are negotiating a change in identity, a loss of intimacy, and sometimes a loss of friends. Widowers go through many of the same experiences, but more widowers remarry than do widows. Big changes late in life can be devastating, making it even more important to watch your health so you're in good shape to handle change.

So as you age, be prepared for changes that might be hard to navigate—and don't try to do it alone. There are many fine organizations and counselors dedicated to aiding people making such transitions.

Cool Fact: At 103 years of age, Kathryn "Kitty" Hodges of Seattle became the oldest tandem skydiver. (Several 102-year-olds had preceded her.) It's never too late to try something new!

What other aging problems start with Y?

Z 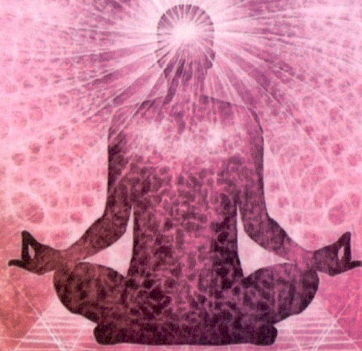 is for Zen

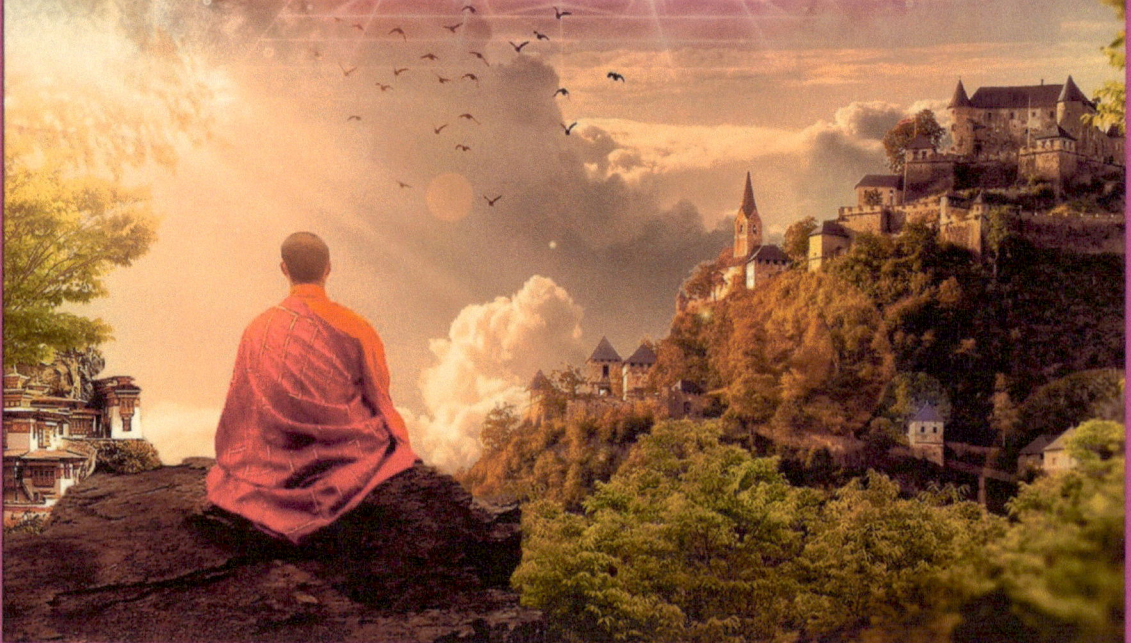

Zen is so simple, that it's virtually impossible to grasp.
—*M.E.*

Z is for **Zen**. Originating in China during the Tang Dynasty, Zen is a Japanese school of Mahayana Buddhism. The Chinese word *ch'an*, from a Sanskrit word meaning "thought," "absorption," or "meditation," is pronounced "Zen" in Japanese. The purpose of Zen is to see things as they are, to observe things as they are, and to let everything go as it goes. Just as we look to our parents for guidance when we are young, and society looks to its elders for good governance, we often look to philosophers or religious leaders to tell us how to act in life. Zen Buddhism turns that search on its head and delivers seemingly contradictory or frivolous answers to the questions that most concern us. The aim is to shock us out of our mundane ways of thinking.

Breathe in, breathe out. Breathe in, breathe out.
Forget this, and attaining enlightenment will be the least of your problems.

Don't get locked into believing there is a right way and a wrong way of looking at life. Garrison Keller, paraphrasing E. Joseph Cossman, said, "As the middle broadens, the mind narrows." But if aging teaches us anything, it is that most of the things that concern us early in life aren't nearly as important as they seemed at the time. Learn to let things go, and you may be surprised what new things open up. Yoko Ono said that "the Zen tradition of doing the thing that is the most embarrassing for you to do and seeing what you come up with and how you deal with it" is the way to find new avenues to explore. Aging does bring challenges we never had before, at just the time when we may feel the least capable of dealing with them. Shuryn Susuki wrote, in *Zen Mind, Beginners Mind: Informal Talks on Zen Meditation*, that "Zen practice is to open up our small minds." Old age is a good time to be open to another way of viewing the world. Who knows, you might even gain enlightenment.

Cool Fact: Shuryn Suzuki, born 1904 in Kanagawa, Japan, was ordained as a novice monk at age 13. He rose through the ranks and at age 22 received Dharma transmission, which establishes one as a "successor in an unbroken lineage of teachers and disciples theoretically traced back to the Buddha himself." In 1959 Suzuki took over the only Soto Zen temple in San Francisco, California. At the time, young American beatniks were discovering Zen, and Suzuki decided he would teach the discipline to Westerners. The group that sat with him eventually formed the San Francisco Zen Center, bought a building in the Lower Haight neighborhood, and turned it into a Zen temple. During this period, Suzuki founded the first Zen Buddhist monastery outside of Asia. His group became one of the most influential Zen organizations in the United States.

What other aging problem starts with Z?

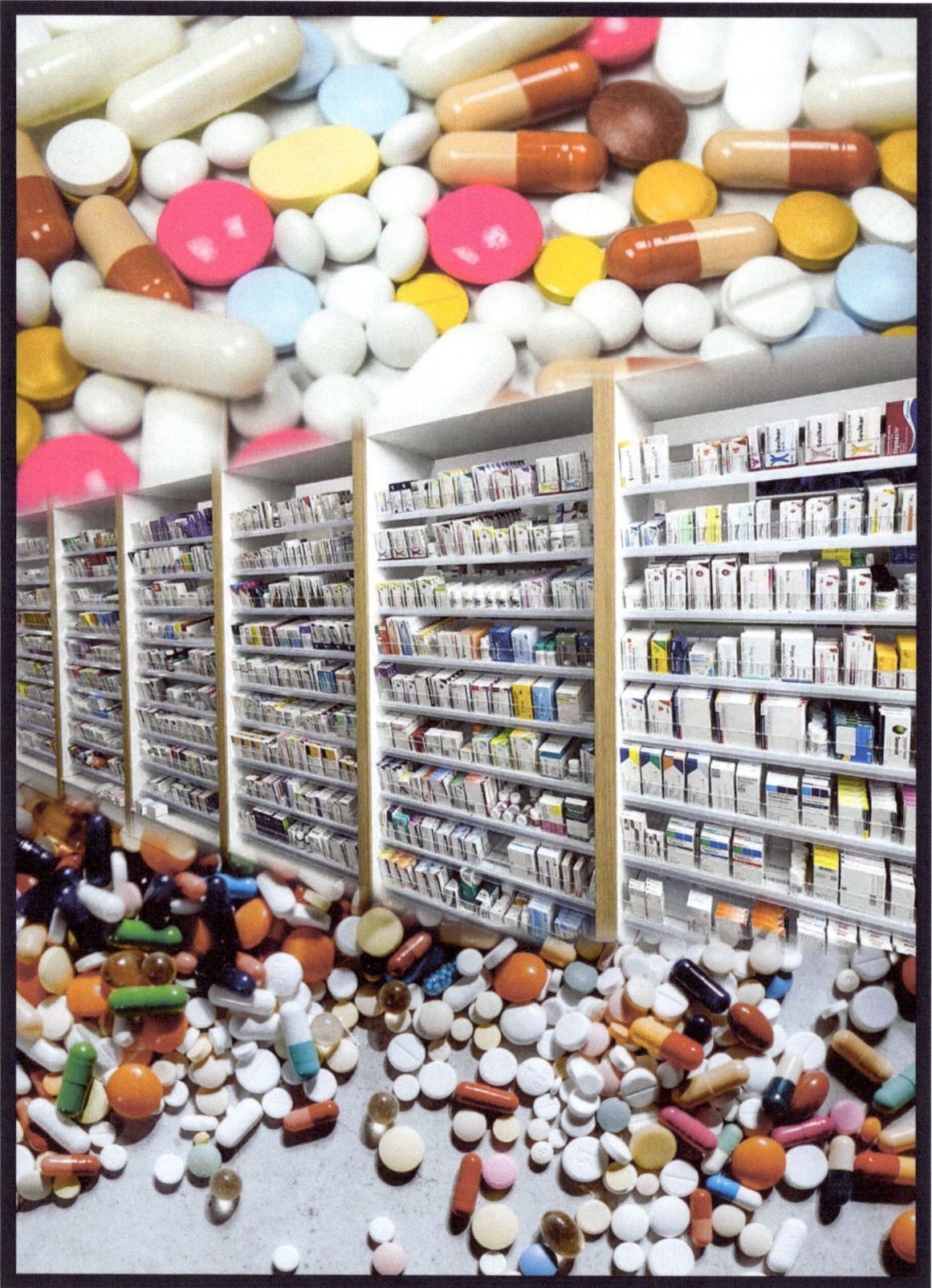

A group of retired classical musicians on medication got together to play music, they call themselves, The Pill harmonic.

—*M.E.*

Disclaimer: **The contents of this book are for information and entertainment purposes only and may not be construed as medical advice or instruction. Readers should consult appropriate health professionals on any matter relating to their health and well-being.**

This disclaimer, or a version of it, will be found on all those sites that show up on your computer claiming to cure your (fill in the blank) in no time. With very little variation—perhaps they are made by the same production company?—each site claims that in the *next few minutes* (or more likely 45 minutes), this sincere, honest-looking man or woman, sometimes dressed in a white coat, will take you through the story of his/her discovery of this miracle cure. Looking right into the camera, and with periodic assurances that the cure will be revealed *at any moment* (and intercut with images of beautiful young women in bikinis or old couples enjoying a walk, riding bicycles, snuggling by the fire, or of people acting out the emotions being described, depending on what is being promoted), the presenter and the story grinds on. The narrator dramatically tells of the discovery that Big Pharma doesn't want you to know about. The healing plant, flower, or obscure herb, to which has been added even more healing treasures, is now available in the form of a capsule! Regardless of the enormous amount of time, effort, and money put into developing it, this won't cost you $1,500.00—even though you would willing pay that much, given how great it is. No! One month's supply is ONLY $69.99! But if you buy three months' supply, it will cost you just $49.99! For six months' supply, *even less* (plus S&H)! Results are *fully guaranteed* but if you are not completely satisfied, simply return the unused bottles for a complete refund, paying only the shipping cost.

Are these miracle cures worth trying? To me, a six-month supply sounds more like long-term care than a cure. But if you have the money, time, and the discipline to return them if they're not working, go ahead.

Cool Fact: A study carried out by Stanford Medicine Investigators has shown that our organs age at different rates. It found that 1 in 5 otherwise healthy adults over 50 is walking around with at least one organ aging at a strongly accelerated rate. Monitoring the health of individual organs may reveal those that are undergoing accelerated aging, making it possible to treat people before they get sick.

More A to Z Aging Issues

A   Asthma, Alzheimer's, angina, ague

B   Bowels, bile, basalioma

C   Cancer, cognition, colitis, colon, carcinoma, cruise ships

D   Diabetes, dentistry, dysphagia

E   Erectile dysfunction, edema, ear hair.

F   Fibrosis, fatigue, fungus

G   Gastrectomy, glaucoma, gingivitis, gout

H   Heart disease, hemorrhoids

I   Insomnia, infections, irritability

J   Jaundice, jaws

K   Kidney failure, keratosis

L   Liver failure, lumbago, Lyme disease

M   Myopia, menopause, melanoma, memory

N   Nephritis, neurosis, nose hair

O   Osteoporosis, orgasm (lack of)

P   Prostate, pancreas, psoriasis, passwords

Q   Quinsy

R   Raynaud's disease, radiation

S   Scoliosis, stroke, sciatica, stenosis

T   Tendonitis, tetanus, teeth

U   Ulcers, UTIs

V   Vision, vascular dementia

W   West Nile virus, whooping cough

X   Xenophobia

Y   Yellow fever

Z   Zika virus

References

Arbott, Stephen, and Mike Haskins. *Man Walks into a Bar.* London: Ebury Press, 2004.

The Editors of FC&A Medical Publishing. *The Country Doctor Handbook.* Peachtree, GA: FC&A Medical Publishing, 2007.

Kunz, Jeffrey, ed. *American Medical Association, Family Medical Guide,* New York: Random House 1982.

Marion, Joseph. *Anti-Aging Manual: The Encyclopedia of Natural Health.* South Woodstock, CT: Information Pioneers, Publisher, 1999. PDF available online at

https://www.scribd.com/document/793090486/Anti-Aging-Manual-Marion-Joseph-B-1999.

Rost, Amy. *Natural Healing Wisdom & Know-How.* New York: Black Dog & Leventhal Publishers, Inc., 2009.

Swerdlow, Joel. *Nature's Medicine.* Washington, D.C.: National Geographic Society, 2000.

And public domain articles from AARP, the Arthritis Foundation, aplaceom.com, Johns Hopkins Medical, National Institute of Neurology Disorders and Strokes, Purehealth, my.clevelandclinic.org, *Men's Health,* Goodnewsnetwork.org, ONE.org, MedicalNewsToday, getsightcare.net, American College of Rheumatology, Texas Health and Human Services, BrainMattersResearch, Wikipedia, pubMedinchi.nim.nih.gov, Elli-Q, thezensite.com, and Stanford Medicine.